Nourishing Recipes

A Gastric Sleeve Cookbook for Healthful Living

Andrew Wilson

Copyright © 2023 - All rights reserved.

TABLE OF CONTENT

INTRODUCTION ____ 1

Before Operation Recipes _____________________________________ 2

Simple Asian Grilled Chicken _____________________________________ 3

Steak Fajitas ____ 5

Chicken with Lemon Garlic Sauce _________________________________ 7

White Chocolate Protein Shake ___________________________________ 9

Vanilla Protein Shake ____ 10

Veggie-Loaded Breakfast Casserole _______________________________ 11

Orange Chicken Lettuce Wrap ____________________________________ 13

Hint of Orange Vanilla Protein Shake ______________________________ 15

Easy Greek Grilled Chicken_______________________________________ 16

15 Minute Garlic Shrimp in Butter Sauce ___________________________ 18

Slow Cooker Barbacoa ____ 20

Baked Salmon with Chimichurri Sauce_____________________________ 22

Brussel Sprout Salad with Ginger Miso Dressing_____________________ 24

Phase One Recipes ____ 26

Chicken Stock ____ 27

Non-Alcoholic Mint Mojito_______________________________________ 29

Peppercorn Chicken Broth _______________________________________ 30

Sugar-Free Strawberry Limeade___________________________________ 31

Rooibos Mint Tea ____ 32

Curried Root Soup ____ 33

Phase Two Recipes____ 35

Oatmeal Cookie Shake ____ 36

Scrambled Eggs with Black Bean Puree _______________________ 37

Frozen Mocha Frappuccino _______________________________ 39

Black Bean and Lime Puree_______________________________ 40

Chocolate PB2 Banana Protein Shake _______________________ 42

Pumpkin Protein Smoothie_______________________________ 43

Apple Cucumber Juice___________________________________ 44

Vitamin C Juice _______________________________________ 45

Cherry Mango Smoothie_________________________________ 46

Coco-Rita Cocktail _____________________________________ 47

5-A-Day Smoothie _____________________________________ 48

Beetroot and Butterbean Hummus _________________________ 49

Strawberry Greek Yogurt Whip ___________________________ 50

Italian Chicken Puree ___________________________________ 51

Oven Baked Ricotta_____________________________________ 52

Pureed Salsa and Beans__________________________________ 53

Egg-Chilada ____ 54

Fat-Free Polenta _______________________________________ 56

Phase Three Recipes __________________________________ 58

Soft Mexican Chicken Salad ______________________________ 59

Peanut Butter Jelly Pancakes _____________________________ 60

High-Protein Pumpkin Pie Oatmeal ________________________ 61

Baked Tomatoes _______________________________________ 62

Classic Hummus_______________________________________ 63

Cheesecake Pudding Recipe ______________________________ 64

Creamy Cauliflower Puree _______________________________ 65

Tuna Salad____ 67

Overnight Oats _______________________________________ 68

Winter Sunshine Smoothie ____ 69

Chocolate Porridge ____ 70

Mugastrone ____ 72

Phase Four Recipes ____ 73

Steak Fajitas ____ 74

Pumpkin and Black Bean Soup ____ 76

Greek Yogurt Chicken ____ 78

Whopper Veggie Burger ____ 79

Brown Rice and Black Bean Casserole ___________________________________ 80

Shrimp Ceviche ____ 82

Taco Beef ____ 84

Slow cooker Chicken Enchiladas _______________________________________ 86

Creamy Green Chile Enchilada Soup ____________________________________ 89

Tilapia Veracruz ____ 92

Taco Pie ____ 95

Slow Cooker Carnitas "Nachos" ____ 97

Chipotle Steak Salad ____ 99

Chile Relleno Casserole ____ 101

Steak and Mushroom Fajita Sandwiches ________________________________ 103

Chili Lime Jalapeno Turkey Burgers ____________________________________ 105

Cilantro Lime Chicken with Tomato Relish _______________________________ 107

Turkey Skillet with Salsa and Eggs _____________________________________ 109

Chicken Chili with Jalapeno and Cheddar ________________________________ 111

Grilled Chicken with Pico de Gallo _____________________________________ 113

Turkey Taco Meatballs ____ 115

Seven Layer Mexican Salad ____ 117

Almond Chicken ____ 120

Autumn Coleslaw ____ 122

Roasted Salmon ____ 124

Steak and Potato Skewers ___________________________________ 126

Easy Pork Stir-Fry ____ 128

Ricotta and Spinach Frittata _________________________________ 130

Puy and Tomato Lentils _____________________________________ 132

Chicken Chili ____ 134

Stuffed Romano Peppers ____________________________________ 136

Weetabix Fruitcake ____ 138

Pink Lady Cornmeal Cake ___________________________________ 140

Chicken Curry ____ 142

Pacific Cod with Fajita Vegetables (Dairy-Free) _________________ 144

Salmon with Summer Salsa (Dairy-Free) _______________________ 146

Cilantro Lime Cauliflower Rice _______________________________ 148

Sweet Pepper Poppers _____________________________________ 149

Roasted Corn Guacamole ___________________________________ 151

Bean and Spinach Burrito ___________________________________ 153

Stuffed Southwest Style Sweet Potatoes _______________________ 155

Vegetable Chili ____ 157

Corn and Black Bean Salad __________________________________ 159

Spicy Peanut Vegetarian Chili ________________________________ 161

Black Bean, Rice, and Zucchini Skillet _________________________ 163

Conclusion ____ 165

Introduction

Welcome to 'Nourishing Recipes: A Gastric Sleeve Cookbook for Healthful Living.' This book is specially crafted to guide you through your nutritional journey following a gastric sleeve surgery. We understand that adjusting to a new way of eating can be complex and, sometimes, a little intimidating. That's why we have devoted careful attention to creating delicious and nutrient-dense recipes that correspond to each stage of your post-operative dietary progression.

Within this cookbook, you will discover a diverse array of dishes designed to meet your specific dietary requirements in each of the five critical phases following surgery – from the initial liquid diet to the eventual transition to solid foods. Regardless of your culinary skill level, these recipes are accessible, easy to prepare, and tailored for a post-gastric sleeve lifestyle.

Remember, eating well after a gastric sleeve surgery isn't just about managing your weight - it's about enjoying your food while nourishing your body. We hope this cookbook serves as an invaluable resource on your journey towards healthful living. Here's to delicious dishes and a healthier you. Enjoy the culinary journey!

Before Operation Recipes

Simple Asian Grilled Chicken

Prep: 5 mins

Cook: 10 mins

Servings – 4

What You Need:

- Ground ginger, 1/2 tsp

- Skinless, boneless chicken breasts, 1.5 lbs

- Pepper, 1/4 tsp

- Light soy sauce, 2 tbs

- Salt, 1/2 tsp

- Mayonnaise, 2 tbs

- Rice vinegar, 2 tbs

- Honey, 1 1/2 tbs

- Sriracha, 1 tbs

- Minced garlic, 2 cloves

What You Do:

1. Start by whisking together the ginger, pepper, salt, mayonnaise, rice vinegar, soy sauce, honey, sriracha, and garlic until smooth. If you want, you can pulse them togetherin a blender.

2. Add the chicken to a zip-top bag and add the marinade. Shake it around to coat the chicken. Let the chicken marinate for at least 30 minutes.

3. Heat up your grill to medium-high. Spray it with some

nonstick spray if needed. Addthe chicken to the grill. Discard the marinade. Cook until the chicken reaches 165 degrees.

4. Serve with a little garnish of cilantro if desired.Calories: 219

Fat: 7.1 g

Protein: 32.4 g

Carb: 4.3 g

Steak Fajitas

Prep: 3 hrs 15 mins

Cook: 15 mins

Servings – 6

What You Need:

- Marinade:
- Chopped cilantro, ¼ cup
- Pepper, ½ tsp
- Minced garlic, 1 tbs
- Salt, 1 tsp
- Paprika, 1 tsp
- Chili powder, 2 tsp
- Red pepper flakes, ½ tsp
- Cumin, 2 tsp
- Olive oil, 3 tbs
- Worcestershire sauce, 2 tbs
- No sugar added pineapple juice, ¼ cup
- Lime juice, ⅓ cup
- Fajitas:
- Bell peppers, 2-3
- Sliced large poblano, 1
- Sliced white onions, 2

- Oil, 1 tbsp

- Skirt steak, 2 lb

What You Do:

1. Mix all of the marinade ingredients together in a shallow bowl. Taste the marinade to see if you need to adjust any of the seasonings. Cover the steak in the marinade and then allow it to sit for at least two to four hours in the fridge. Take the steak out 30 minutes before cooking.

2. Place a cast iron skillet on high heat. Put in the steak and fry for three to five minutes on each side. Three minutes will put it at medium rare. Reduce the heat of the pan if you need to. Take out the cooked steak and let it rest for a bit before slicing. Slice against the grain into thin slices.

3. Add the rest of the oil to the skillet and add in the peppers, poblano, and onion. Toss the veggies around and cook for a couple of minutes, or until soft. Season with some pepper and salt.

4. Serve in rice bowls or on tortillas, or enjoy it as is.

Calories: 361

Fat: 24.2 g

Protein: 24.5 g

Carb: 13.1 g

Chicken with Lemon Garlic Sauce

Prep: 10 mins

Cook: 20 mins

Servings – 4

What You Need:

- Chopped parsley, 2 tbs
- Heavy cream, ¼ cup
- Red pepper flakes, ½ tsp
- Salted butter, 2 tbs
- Lemon juice, 2 tbsp
- Diced shallots, ⅓ cup
- Olive oil, 1 tbs
- Minced garlic, 1 tbs
- Chicken broth, 1 cup
- Pepper
- Salt
- Skinless, boneless chicken breasts, 4

What You Do:

1. Pound the chicken to half inch thickness. Sprinkle the chicken with pepper and salt.

2. Mix together the red pepper flakes, garlic, lemon juice, and chicken broth.

3. Place your oven rack on the lower third holder and at 375

degrees.

4. Add olive oil to a skillet and put in the chicken. Let it cook for two to three minuteson each side. The chicken doesn't have to be fully cooked at this point. Set aside.

5. Lower the heat and add in the shallots with the chicken broth mixture. Deglaze the pan. Up the heat and allow the sauce to simmer and cook for 10 to 15 minutes, or untilthere is about a third of a cup of the sauce.

6. Once thickened, take it off the heat and stir in the butter until completely melted. Whisk in the heavy cream. Set it back on the heat, but don't let it boil. Add the chickenback in and coat it with the sauce. Slide it into the oven and cook for five to eight minutes, or until the chicken has cooked through.

7. Top with the parsley.

Calories: 302

Fat: 16.1 g

Protein: 33.9 g

Carb: 4.6 g

White Chocolate Protein Shake

Prep: 0 mins

Cook: 3 mins

Servings – 1

What You Need:

- Sugar-free white chocolate pudding mix, ½ tbs
- Vanilla whey protein powder, 1 scoop
- Ice cubes, 6
- Unsweetened almond milk, 8 oz

What You Do:

1. Add all of the ingredients to your blender and mix them together until it is completely smooth.

Calories: 295

Fat: 3 g

Protein: 23 g

Carb: 10 g

Vanilla Protein Shake

Prep: 0 mins

Cook: 3 mins

Servings – 1

What You Need:

- Dash of nutmeg
- Unflavored whey protein powder, ½ scoop
- Vanilla whey protein powder, ½ scoop
- Ice cubes, 6
- Unsweetened vanilla almond milk, 6 oz

What You Do:

1. Add all of the ingredients to your blender and mix them together until it is completely smooth. Sprinkle some nutmeg over tops if desired.

Calories: 295

Fat: 3 g

Protein: 24 g

Carb: 5 g

Veggie-Loaded Breakfast Casserole

Prep: 20 mins

Cook: 45 mins

Servings – 10-12

What You Need:

- Shredded cheese, 1 cup
- Pepper
- Salt
- Hot sauce, ¼ cup Half and half, ⅓ cup
- Eggs, 10
- Shredded potatoes, 20 oz
- Baby spinach, 2 cups
- Diced bell pepper, 2
- Diced red onion, ½
- Minced garlic, 2 tsp
- Sliced mushrooms, 8-10
- Oil, 2 tbs

What You Do:

1. Place a tablespoon of oil in a large skillet on medium. Put the mushrooms in and let them cook for four minutes, or until they begin to brown up. Add a bit of salt, garlic, and onions and allow them to cook for two minutes. Set everything aside in a plate. Add in the remaining oil and cook the peppers for a minute. Place in the baby spinach

and cook until wilted. Set aside.

2. Spray a nine by 13-inch baking dish with nonstick spray. Spread the shredded potatoes in the bottom. Try to get them as even as possible. Add all of the veggies overthe potatoes and set aside.

3. Place the rack in the middle of your oven and set to 375 degrees.

4. Add the hot sauce, half and half, egg, pepper, and salt in a large bowl and whisk it all together. Pour this over the veggies and top everything with the cheese. Season again.

5. Slide this into the oven and cook uncovered for 45 to 50 minutes. The eggs should be set and the cheese golden brown. Let this rest for around ten minutes before slicing.

Calories: 172

Fat: 9.9 g

Protein: 9.3 g

Carb: 11.6 g

Orange Chicken Lettuce Wrap

Prep: 5 mins

Cook: 15 mins

Servings – 10-12

What You Need:

- Orange Sauce:
- Water, 2 tbs
- Soy sauce, 2 tbs
- Cornstarch, ½ tbs
- Red pepper flakes, ½ tsp
- Ginger, ½ tsp
- Minced garlic, 1 tsp
- Brown sugar, ¼ cup
- Apple cider vinegar, 2 tbs
- Orange zest, 1 tbsp
- Orange juice, ½ cup
- Chicken Filling:
- Sesame seeds, lettuce leaves, and scallions – topping
- Mandarin oranges, 10.5 oz
- Minced garlic, 2 tsp
- Ground chicken, 1 lb
- Oil, 1 tbsp

What You Do:

6. Place all of the sauce ingredients into a mason jar. Cover and shake really well untilthe ingredients are well mixed.

7. Pour your sauce into a saucepan and let it heat up on medium. Once the sauce starts tosimmer, lower the heat, and let it cook for a couple of minutes. The sauce should be ableto coat a spoon. Remove from heat and cool.

8. Add the oil in and let it heat up. Add in the ground chicken and break it up intosmaller lumps with a wooden spoon.

9. Add in the garlic and allow this to cook for five to seven minutes, or until the chickenhas cooked all the way.

10. Drizzle the sauce over the chicken and cook for another one to two minutes. Add insome pepper and salt.

11. Let the filling cool for a moment before filling the lettuce leaves. Top the filling withsesame seeds and orange slices once you fill the lettuce leaves.

Calories: 112

Fat: 4.9 g

Protein: 8.6 g

Carb: 8.5 g

Hint of Orange Vanilla Protein Shake

Prep: 5 mins

Cook: 0 mins

Servings – 1

What You Need:

- Ice cubs, 6

- Mandarin orange juice, 1 tbs

- Vanilla whey protein powder, 1 scoop

- 2% cottage cheese, 2 tbs

- Unsweetened almond milk, 6 oz

What You Do:

1. Place all of the shake ingredients in your blender and mix it together until it issmooth.

Calories: 250

Fat: 2 g

Protein: 24 g

Carb: 5 g

Easy Greek Grilled Chicken

Prep: 5 mins

Cook: 10 mins

Servings – 4

What You Need:

- Red wine vinegar, 1 tbs
- Olive oil, 3 tbs
- Minced garlic, 1 tbs
- Chopped rosemary, ½ tsp
- Cayenne pepper, ¼ tsp
- Fresh lemon juice, 3 tbs
- Fresh thyme, 1 tsp
- Dried oregano, ½ tsp
- Pepper, ½ tsp
- Salt, ½ tsp
- Skinless, boneless chicken breasts, 1.5 l

What You Do:

2. Using a small bowl, whisk together the minced garlic, salt, lemon juice, pepper, oliveoil, rosemary, red wine vinegar, oregano, cayenne, and thyme.

3. Lay the chicken breasts in a large zip-top baggie and pour in the marinade you just mixed up. Zip up the bag and shake it all together until the chicken has been coated. Let the chicken marinade for at least ten minutes. The longer it

marinates, the more flavor the chicken will have.

4. Heat your grill, either indoor or outdoor. Spritz the grates with some cooking spray ifneeded. Lay the chicken on the grill and get rid of any leftover marinade. Allow the chicken to cook for five to six minutes on each side, or until it has reached an internal temperature of 165 degrees.

5. Serve with a garnish of chopped parsley if desired.Calories: 191

Fat: 5.5 g

Protein: 32.1 g

Carb: 1.4 g

15 Minute Garlic Shrimp in Butter Sauce

Prep: 10 mins

Cook: 5 mins

Servings – 4

What You Need:

- PepperSalt
- Cubed butter, 3 tbs
- Minced garlic, 6-8 cloves
- Chopped parsley, ¼ cup
- Caper brine, 1 tbs
- Lemon juice, 2 tbs
- Cleaned shrimp, 1 lb
- Red pepper flakes, ½ tsp
- Olive oil, 1 tbs

What You Do:

1. Place a skillet on high heat and allow it to heat up. Add in the red pepper flakes and olive oil and let them cook together for about 30 seconds. This infuses the red pepper flakes into the oil.

2. Place the shrimp in the pan and spread them out so that they can cook evenly. Allow them to cook for around a minute. Flip them as needed. Add in the caper bring, lemon

3. juice and garlic and let this cook for a minute more.

4. Add in half of the parsley and the cubed butter. Swirl the pan so that the butter will start to melt slowly. Let it cook for about two to three minutes or until the butter melts.

5. As the butter melts, it will start to make a thick sauce. Add in the rest of parsley and mix together. The shrimp need to turn opaque. If the sauce starts to thicken up too much,you can take the shrimp out and add in a teaspoon of water to thin the sauce to a pourable consistency.

6. This recipe is only meant to make enough of a sauce to coat the shrimp, but it is flavorful enough to serve along with some pasta or rice that has been tossed in olive oil ifyou want.

Calories: 190

Fat: 13.3 g

Protein: 15.7 g

Carb: 1.8 g

Slow Cooker Barbacoa

Prep: 10 mins

Cook: 4 hrs 10 mins

Servings – 10-12

What You Need:

- Sliced onion, ½ medium
- Bay leaves, 2
- Pepper, 1 tsp
- Oil, 1 tbs
- Tomato paste, 1 tbs
- Salt, 1 tsp
- Ground cloves, ¼ tsp
- Oregano, 2 ½ tsp
- Cumin, 4 tsp
- Beef broth, ½ cup Lime juice, 2 tbs
- Chipotle peppers, 2
- Garlic, 5 cloves
- Apple cider vinegar, 3 tbs
- Fat trimmed chuck roast cut into 2-inch pieces, 3 lb

What You Do:

1. Add the pepper, salt, oil, tomato paste, cloves, oregano, cumin, beef broth, lime juice,chipotle peppers, garlic, and apple cider vinegar in a blender and mix together until

smooth.

2. Place the beef, sliced onion, and bay leaves in your slow cooker.

3. Pour the sauce you made in step one over the beef. Toss everything together to combine. Place the lid on the cooker and set on low for six to eight hours. If you want itto cook faster, you can set it to high for three to four hours. The beef should be tender and falling apart.

4. Take out the bay leaves. Using two forks, shred the beef up into smaller pieces. Tossthe beef back in the juices. Place the lid back on and let it cook for another ten to 15 minutes so that the beef soaks up all the juices.

5. Serve the beef however you would like.

Calories: 180

Fat: 7.7 g

Protein: 24.8 g

Carb: 3.4 g

Baked Salmon with Chimichurri Sauce

Prep: 5 mins

Cook: 15 mins

Servings – 4

What You Need:

- Red pepper flakes, ¼ tsp
- Lime juice, 1 tbs
- Cilantro leaves, 2 tbs
- Parsley, ½ cup
- Chopped scallions, 2
- Red wine vinegar, 1 tbs
- Pepper
- Salt
- Minced garlic, 3 cloves
- Olive oil, ¼ cup + 1 tbs
- Salmon, 1.25 lb

What You Do:

1. Take the salmon out of the fridge and let it sit at room temperature for at least 15 minutes before you cook it. Place the rack in the middle of your oven and heat to 375 degrees.

2. Lay the salmon on a section of tin foil that is large enough

fold over and seal up.

3. With a brush, brush the fish with a tablespoon of olive oil and sprinkle it with some pepper and salt as well as one minced garlic cloves. Cover the salmon with foil and sealit up so that everything is enclosed.

4. Slide the fish into the oven and let it cook for 12 to 14 minutes, or until it is firm andflakes easily. As the salmon is cooking, fix the salmon. Depending on how thick your salmon fillet is, you may need to cook it for a bit longer.

5. For the sauce, add a quarter of a teaspoon of pepper, a half teaspoon of salt, red pepper flakes, lime juice, red wine vinegar, cilantro, parsley, scallions, remaining garlic,and a quarter cup of olive oil to a food processor and pulse it until it forms a thick sauce.

6. Once the salmon has finished cooking, take it out of the oven and spread a tablespoonof sauce over the top. Place it back in the oven and allow it to broil for two to three minutes. Make sure that the fish does not burn. Take it out of the oven and serve it with the rest of the sauce.

Calories: 456

Fat: 36 g

Protein: 29.6 g

Carb: 2.6 g

Brussel Sprout Salad with Ginger Miso Dressing

Prep: 15 mins

Cook: 15 mins

Servings – 4-6

What You Need:

Dressing:

- Honey, 2 tbs
- White miso paste, 1 ½ tbs
- Low-sodium soy sauce, 1 tbs
- Sesame oil, 1 tbs
- Rice vinegar, 1 tbs
- Grated ginger, 1 tbs
- Lime juice, 2 tbs
- Canola oil, 2 tbs

Salad:

- Wonton strips and sesame seeds (serving)
- Chopped peanuts, ½ cup
- Sliced Serrano pepper
- Cooked shredded chicken, 1 ½ cups
- Thinly sliced scallions, 4
- Chopped cilantro, ½ cup

- Shaved Brussel sprouts and chopped kale, 7-8 cups

What You Do:

1. Place all of the dressing ingredients into a blender and pulse until smooth. You canalso just whisk it all together in a bowl.

2. Toss all of the salad ingredients together and drizzle the salad with the dressing. Tosseverything to combine.

3. Serve the salad with some wonton strips and sesame seeds. Calories: 234

Fat: 14.8 g

Protein: 13.1 g

Carb: 15.8 g

Phase One Recipes

Chicken Stock

Chicken Stock

Prep: 10 mins

Cook: 5-6 hrs

Servings – 16

What You Need:

- Water to fill the potLemon, 2 slices
- Apple cider vinegar, 1 tbs
- Peppercorns, ½ tsp
- Sea salt, 2 tsp
- Parsley, 5 stems
- Thyme, 3-5 sprigs
- Bay leaf
- Garlic cloves, 4-5
- Celery stalks, 2
- Peeled carrots, 2
- Quartered onion, 1
- Whole chicken

What You Do:

1. Place a six to eight quart pot with a tight lid on a stovetop. Clean the chicken, makingsure there is nothing inside of it.

2. Add all of the ingredients to your pot and add enough water into it to cover everything. Place on the lid, making sure it

fits tightly, and allow it to come to a boil. Turn the heat down and let it simmer for four hours.

3. If using a whole chicken, remove the meat after two hours so that it doesn't overcookand add the bones back into the pot.

4. You can save the meat for later use.

5. The pot should stay covered so that the liquid doesn't evaporate.

6. Once cooked, strain through a mesh colander. Discard everything except for theliquid.

7. Allow the stock to come to room temperature and then store in quart containers in thefridge for three days, or you can freeze it for six months.

Calories: 10

Fat: .6 g

Protein: .7 g

Carb: .7 g

Non-Alcoholic Mint Mojito

Prep: 3 mins

Cook: 30 mins

Servings – 1

What You Need:

- Lime juice, 1 oz
- Fresh mint leaves, ½ cup
- Natural sweetener, ½ cup
- Water, 2 cups

What You Do:

1. Place the water and sweetener in a pot and allow it to boil for around five minutes, or until it has thickened into a syrup.

2. Place the mint leaves in a glass jar and pour in the syrup. Cover the jar and allow it to steep for at least 20 minutes. You can use this now, or you can save it for later.

3. Place ice in a glass and pour in a tablespoon of the syrup and a half cup of cold water. Add in the lime juice and mix everything together.

4. You can adjust the syrup and lime juice to your preference. Calories: 32

Fat: 0 g

Protein: 0 g

Carb: 3 g

Peppercorn Chicken Broth

Prep: 2 mins

Cook: 20 mins

Servings – 2

What You Need:

- Peppercorns, 1 tbs

- Chicken broth, 2 cups

What You Do:

1. Place both ingredients in a pot and turn it to high heat until it starts to boil.

2. Lower the heat down to a simmer and let it cook for 20 minutes.

3. Take the pot off the heat and then strain out the peppercorns. Allow this to cool andthen sip when needed.

Calories: 10

Fat: .6 g

Protein: .7 g

Carb: .7 g

Sugar–Free Strawberry Limeade

Prep: 0 mins

Cook: 3 mins

Servings – 1

What You Need:

- Ice cubes, 6

- Strawberry extract, ½ tsp

- Cold water, 1 ½ cups

- Juice of half a lime

What You Do:

1. Mix together the strawberry extract, lime juice, and water. Add the ice cubes to a cup and pour in the strawberry mixture. If you want, you can sweeten with a calorie-free sweetener.

Calories: 12

Fat: 0 g

Protein: .1 g

Carb: 2.1 g

Rooibos Mint Tea

Prep: 3 mins

Cook: 30 mins

Servings – 6

What You Need:

- Boiling water, 1 gallon
- Sweetener, 1-2 tbsp (don't sweeten if you have just had your surgery)
- Fresh mint, 2 tbs
- Sliced lemon
- Rooibos tea, 6 bags

What You Do:

2. Place the water on high heat. After it has started boiling, turn the heat off and add inthe tea bags.
3. Pour into a pitcher and mix in everything else. Place the pitcher in the sunlight andallow the tea to steep for at least 30 minutes.
4. Serve over ice.

Calories: 4

Fat: 0 g

Protein: .2 g

Carb: 1.4 g

Curried Root Soup

Prep: 10 mins

Cook: 50 mins

Servings – 4

What You Need:

- A squeeze of lemon juice
- Vegetable stock, 5 cups
- Curry powder, 1 tsp
- Crushed garlic, 2 cloves
- Pepper
- Salt
- Chopped carrots, 1 lb
- Chopped rutabaga, 1 lb
- Sliced leeks, 2
- Chopped onion
- Cooking spray

What You Do:

1. Give a large skillet a generous spritz of cooking spray and allow it to heat up. Add in the carrots, rutabaga, leeks, and onions along with a sprinkling of pepper and salt. Allowthis to fry up for around 30 minutes, stirring occasionally. Add some water or a little more cooking spray if the pan starts to look dry. The vegetables need to soften up, but they should not take on a deep color.

2. Add in the curry powder and garlic, allowing this to cook for one to two minutes.

3. Mix in the stock and allow everything to come to a boil. Lower the heat down and letit simmer for 15 minutes.

4. Once cooked, add batches to a blender and puree until smooth. You can also use animmersion blender if you have one.

5. Place back in the pan and add in a squeeze of lemon juice. Check the seasonings andadjust if needed. Serve with some yogurt, mint leaves, or mango chutney if you would like.

Calories: 125

Fat: 2.5 g

Protein: 4.5 g

Carb: 22.3 g

Phase Two Recipes

Oatmeal Cookie Shake

Prep: 5 mins

Cook: 0 mins

Servings – 1

What You Need:

- Vanilla extract, ¼ tsp
- Oatmeal, 1 tbs
- Ground cinnamon, ½ tsp
- Low-fat nut milk, 1 cup
- Vanilla whey protein powder, 1 scoop

What You Do:

1. Add the vanilla, oatmeal, cinnamon, milk, and protein powder to a blender. Mixeverything together. If you want your shake to be thicker, you can add some ice.

2. Pour the shake into a glass. If you want, you can serve it with a dusting of cinnamon,a couple of nuts, or a squirt of low-fat cream.

Calories: 179

Fat: 5.1 g

Protein: 23.5 g

Carb: 8.3 g

Scrambled Eggs with Black Bean Puree

Prep: 5 mins

Cook: 10 mins

Servings – 1

What You Need:

- Black Bean Pure:
- Unflavored whey protein powder, 1 tbs
- Vegetable or chicken broth, 2 tbs
- Green enchilada sauce, 3 tbs
- Rinsed black beans, ½ cupEgg:
- Pepper, pinchSalt, pinch Egg

What You Do:

1. Black Bean Puree:
2. After you have rinsed off your black beans, add them to a small pot and let them heatover medium.
3. Add in two and a half tablespoons of the enchilada sauce to your beans and stir themtogether. Allow the mixture to cook for another two minutes.
4. Mix in the chicken broth.
5. Add the black bean mixture to your blender and mix it until completely smooth.
6. Make sure you are careful because the mixture is hot.

7. If you have an immersion blender you can use that as well to puree the beans.

8. Pour the pureed beans into a bowl.

9. Allow the pureed beans to cool slightly and then mix in the protein powder until wellcombined.

10. Cover them to keep them warm until you have cooked your egg.

11. Refrigerate whatever you have left over.

12. Egg:

13. Heat a pan on medium high, and as it is warming, whisk the egg together with the pepper and salt until it is well incorporated.

14. Pour the mixed egg into the hot pan. With a rubber spatula, slowly scramble the eggsuntil cooked all the way through.

15. Once the egg is nearly cooked, but it still has a liquid texture, fold it onto itself andthen place it on a plate.

16. Top your egg with a tablespoon of the black bean puree you made earlier and thenpour the remaining green enchilada sauce on top.

Calories: 308

Fat: 5.2 g

Protein: 42.9 g

Carb: 22.6 g

Frozen Mocha Frappuccino

Prep: 5 mins

Cook: 0 mins

Servings – 1

What You Need:

- Low-sugar chocolate syrup (optional)
- Low-fat whipped cream (optional)
- Ice, 1 cup
- Cocoa powder, 1 tbs
- Liquid sweetener, 3-4 drops
- 0% fat Greek yogurt, ½ cup
- Unsweetened almond milk, ¼ cup
- Brewed coffee, ¼ cup

What You Do:

1. Add the ice, cocoa, sweetener, yogurt, milk, and coffee to your blender and pulse it a few times to mix everything together extremely well.

2. Pour your Frappuccino into a tall glass and top it with some whipped cream and chocolate syrup if desired. Enjoy.

Calories: 93

Fat: 2.7 g

Protein: 11.8 g

Carb: 4.84 g

Black Bean and Lime Puree

Prep: 5 mins

Cook: 10 mins

Serving – 1

What You Need:

- Unflavored protein powder, 1 tbs
- Vegetable or chicken broth, ¼ cup
- Jarred jalapeno juice, ½ tbs
- Lime juice, ½ tbs
- Rinsed black beans, ¼ cup

What You Do:

1. After you have rinsed your black beans, place them into a small pot and allow them toheat over medium.

2. Mix in the juice from the jalapenos and the lime juice. Stir everything together andallow it to heat through.

3. Once heated, mix in the chicken broth.

4. Pour the mixture into the blender and mix until it is completely smooth. Be carefulbecause the mixture is hot, and make sure that you hold the lid.

5. If you have an immersion blender, you can use that as well. Pour the mixture into abowl.

6. Allow the mixture to cool slightly and then mix in the protein powder until it is wellmixed.

7. Enjoy.Calories: 180

Fat: 1.9 g

Protein: 30.6 g

Carb: 11.6 g

Chocolate PB2 Banana Protein Shake

Prep: 10 mins

Cook: 0 mins

Servings – 2

What You Need:

- Ice cubes, 4-5
- Frozen sliced banana
- Chocolate whey isolate protein powder, ¼ cup
- PB2 powder, ¼ cup
- Light soy milk, 1 cup

What You Do:

1. Place all of the ingredients in a high-speed blender and mix until everything is smoothand creamy.

Calories: 319

Fat: 4.9 g

Protein: 40.8 g

Carb: 32.6 g

Pumpkin Protein Smoothie

Prep: 5 mins

Cook: 5 mins

Servings – 2

What You Need:

- Ice cubes, 1 cup
- Pumpkin pie spice, ¼ tsp
- Cinnamon, ¼ tsp
- Vanilla whey protein powder, ¼ cup
- Pumpkin puree, ⅓ cup
- Soy milk, ¾ cup
- Vanilla Greek frozen yogurt, ½ cup
- Frozen banana

What You Do:

2. Place all of the ingredients into your blender and mix on high for around two to threeminutes, or until it is smooth. Scrape the sides down as needed.

3. Add a little extra milk if your mixture is too thick. If it's too thin, add extra ice cubes.

Calories: 254

Fat: 3.7 g

Protein: 27.9 g

Carb: 28.7 g

Apple Cucumber Juice

Prep: 5 mins

Cook: 0 mins

Servings – 4

What You Need:

- Head romaine lettuce

- Small mandarin oranges, 3

- Lime

- Large lemon Large cucumber

- Medium apples, 3

What You Do:

1. You will need a juicer for this recipe.

2. Wash all of the fruits and veggies very well. This is because you are going to be usingthe skins as well.

3. Run the fruits and veggies through your juice. This makes 32 ounces of juice.

Calories: 146

Fat: .8 g

Protein: 2 g

Carb: 38.4 g

Vitamin C Juice

Prep: 5 mins

Cook: 0 mins

Servings – 4

What You Need:

- Handful of ginger
- Pineapple, ¼ Limes, 2
- Lemon, 1
- Grapefruits, 5

What You Do:

1. Remove the tops and bottoms from the grapefruits. With a sharp knife, cut around the edges of the peeling. Make sure you don't cut away the pith. This holds a lot of nutrients.Do the same thing with the lemon, limes, and pineapple. If you have a high-quality juicer, you don't have to worry about peeling the lemon and lime.

2. Juice the grapefruits, ginger, limes, and lemon. Lastly, juice the pineapple.

3. Serve over ice and enjoy.Calories: 88

Fat: .4 g

Protein: 1.7 g

Carb: 23.6 g

Cherry Mango Smoothie

Prep: 10 mins

Cook: 5 mins

Servings – 1

What You Need:

- Water, ¾ cup
- Frozen mango, 1 cup
- Water, ½ cup
- Frozen sweeten cherries, 1 cup

What You Do:

1. Allow the mangoes and cherries to sit in separate bowls until they are thawed, which should take around ten minutes.

2. Add the cherries to a blender with half a cup of water and blend until smooth. Add ina little more water if it seems too thick. Pour the mixture into a glass.

3. Rinse out the blender and add in the mango and remaining water. Blend until smooth,adding more water if you need to. Pour this over the cherries and enjoy.

Calories: 185

Fat: 0 g

Protein: 2 g

Carb: 46 g

Coco-Rita Cocktail

Prep: 5 mins

Cook: 0 mins

Servings – 1

What You Need:

- Squeezed orange juice, 2 tbs

- Coconut water, 4 tbs

- Healthy sugar replacement, 2 tbs

- Lime juice, 5 tbs

- Rock salt

- Wedge of lime

What You Do:

1. Get a martini glass and run a wedge of lime around the edge, then dip the glass in salt.

2. Add the orange juice, coconut water, syrup, and lime juice to a shaker and shakevigorously for about 20 seconds.

3. Add ice to your martini glass and strain the drink over the ice. Serve with a limewedge and edible flower if desired.

Calories: 24

Fat: .1 g

Protein: .4 g

Carb: 5.7 g

5–A–Day Smoothie

Prep: 5 mins

Cook: 0 mins

Servings – 2

What You Need:

- Orange juice, ⅔ cup
- Chopped and peeled avocado, ¼
- Low-fat coconut milk, 5 tbs
- Spinach leaves, a small handful
- Dessert pear, 1
- Apple, 1

What You Do:

1. Core the pear and apple and dice them into small chunks.
2. Add them to the blender along with the orange juice, avocado, coconut milk, andspinach. Pulse the mixture until everything is evenly mixed and smooth.
3. Pour into a glass and enjoy.

Calories: 283

Fat: 12.5 g

Protein: 3.2 g

Carb: 40.8 g

Beetroot and Butterbean Hummus

Prep: 5 mins

Cook: 5 mins

Servings – 6

What You Need:

- Pepper
- Extra virgin olive oil, 1 tbsSalt
- Fat-free Greek yogurt, 2 tbs
- Bunch of chopped chives
- Crushed garlic, 1-2 cloves
- Rinsed and drained butterbeans, 14 oz
- Cooked beetroot, 8 oz

What You Do:

1. Dice up the beetroot into small cubes.
2. Place the butterbeans in a food processor along with the pepper, salt, yogurt, oil,chives, and garlic. Blitz everything together until well mixed.
3. Fold the diced beetroot through the mixture.
4. Serve with some crudités.

Calories: 80

Fat: 2.6 g

Protein: 4.2 g

Carb: 10.4 g

Strawberry Greek Yogurt Whip

Prep: 10 mins

Cook: 0 mins

Servings – 6

What You Need:

- Light whipped topping, ½ cup
- Natural no-cal sweetener, 1 tbs
- Fat-free Greek yogurt, ⅔ cup
- Frozen strawberries, 3

What You Do:

1. Add the strawberries to a bowl and allow them to defrost for 60 seconds.
2. Dice up the strawberries until they are well chopped and slightly runny. Add theGreek yogurt and mix together.
3. Add in the sweetener and mix well. Fold the whipped topping into the yogurt mixture.Enjoy this immediately or cover and it and refrigerate it until later.

Calories: 28

Fat: 1 g

Protein: 2 g

Carb: 3 g

Italian Chicken Puree

Prep: 5 mins

Cook: 0 mins

Servings – 1

What You Need:

- Italian seasoning, 1 tsp

- Pepper

- Salt

- Tomato sauce, 1 ½ tbs

- Canned chicken, ¼ cup

What You Do:

1. Add all of the ingredients to your blender and pulse until well mixed and incorporated. You can also use the back of a fork to blend everything together.

2. Place everything in a bowl and microwave it for 30 seconds.

Calories: 73

Fat: 4 g

Protein: 13 g

Carb: 3 g

Oven Baked Ricotta

Prep: 10 mins

Cook: 20 mins

Servings – 4

What You Need:

- Dijon mustard, 1 tsp

- Ground thyme, 1 tsp

- Egg

- 2% cheddar cheese, ¼ cup

- Reduced-fat parmesan, ¼ cup

- Low-fat ricotta cheese, ½ cup

What You Do:

1. Set oven for 400 degrees.

2. Add all of the ingredients to a bowl and mix everything together until well combined.The mixture will look a little gritty and brown but should be smooth.

3. Using a cookie scoop, divide your mixture into four muffin tin cups.

4. Slide this into the oven and let it cook for 20 minutes. Allow to cool slightly beforeserving.

Calories: 69

Fat: 4 g

Protein: 8 g

Carb: 4 g

Pureed Salsa and Beans

Prep: 5 mins

Cook: 10 mins

Servings – 4

What You Need:

- Unflavored whey protein powder, 1 scoop

- Chicken broth, 2 tbs

- Salsa of choice, 2 tbs

- Pinto beans, 15 oz

What You Do:

1. Place all of the ingredients into a small pot and allow it to heat up over medium-high.

2. Make sure you stir it occasionally until everything has warmed through.

3. Pour the mixture into a blender.

4. Puree the mixture for a few minutes until it becomes completely smooth. Be carefulbecause the mixture will be hot.

5. Transfer the pureed food to a serving dish.

6. Divide your leftovers into single-serving containers for easier consumption later.

Calories: 95

Fat: .4 g

Protein: 11.2 g

Carb: 12.2 g

Egg-Chilada

Prep: 5 mins

Cook: 5 mins

Servings – 1

What You Need:

- Fat-free Greek yogurt, 2 tbs

- Shredded Mexican blend cheese, 1 tbs

- Salsa, 2 tbs

- Tofu, 1 ounce

- Salt

- Pepper

- Egg white

- Egg

What You Do:

1. Beat both the whole egg and the egg white together in a small bowl.

2. Add some nonstick spray to a pan and allow it to get heated over medium. Add thebeaten egg to the heated pan, and let it spread out into a circular shape.

3. Let the egg cook on its own for a minute or so until the edges have set up. Sprinklethe top with a bit of salt and pepper as it is cooking.

4. Ease a spatula under the egg and then flip it over. There will probably be some eggthat pours off, but it's not a big deal.

5. Allow the other side of the egg to cook for another minute or so, or until it has cookedall the way through.

6. Down the center of the egg, place the crumbled tofu and cheese. Roll it up like atortilla to form your egg-chilada. Add the yogurt and salsa on top.

Calories: 283

Fat: 14.7 g

Protein: 29 g

Carb: 9.6 g

Fat–Free Polenta

Prep: 5 mins

Cook: 25 mins

Servings – 8

What You Need:

- Chicken broth, 1 cup
- Fat-free milk, 2 cups
- Cornmeal, 1 cup

What You Do:

1. Add the broth and milk to a medium-sized pot and allow to come to a boil.
2. Make sure you stir the mixture continuously.
3. Once it has reached a gentle boil, whisk in the cornmeal.
4. Continue to stir the mixture for another five minutes.
5. Take the mixture off the heat and spread it into an eight by eight-inch casserole dishor a loaf pan.
6. If you prefer your polenta soft, cover it now and allow it to chill.
7. If you would like to firm up your polenta, slide it into a 350-degree oven and allow itto bake for 14 minutes.
8. Once cooked, allow it to cool and then slice it into servings.

Calories: 57

Fat: .4 g

Protein: 3.4 g

Carb: 9.8 g

Phase Three Recipes

Soft Mexican Chicken Salad

Prep: 5 mins

Cook: 5 mins

Servings – 2

What You Need:

- Juice from jarred salsa, 2 tsp

- Taco seasoning, 1 tsp

- Light mayonnaise, 1 tbs

- Canned chicken, drained, 1 cup

What You Do:

1. Put the drained chicken in a bowl. Take a fork and break the chicken into smallpieces.

2. Add the mayonnaise to the chicken and combine well. Mash the chicken into themayonnaise with the fork.

3. Add the salsa juice and taco seasoning into chicken mixture and continue to mash until everything is well combined. Serve and enjoy.

Calories: 180

Fat: 4.8

Protein: 21.9

Carb: 10.9 g

Peanut Butter Jelly Pancakes

Prep: 5 mins

Cook: 10 mins

Servings – 4

What You Need:

- Frozen mixed berries
- Egg whites, 4
- Powdered peanuts, 2 tbs
- Instant oatmeal, ½ cup
- Low-fat cottage cheese, ½ cup

What You Do:

1. Place the egg whites, powdered peanuts, oatmeal, and cottage cheese into a
2. blender and mix until it creates a smooth batter.
3. Pour this mixture into a bowl and then fold in the berry mix.
4. Spritz a skillet with cooking spray. Divide the batter into four pancakes. Oncecooked, enjoy.

Calories: 90

Fat: 1.5 g

Protein: 10 g

Carb: 9 g

High–Protein Pumpkin Pie Oatmeal

Prep: 5 mins

Cook: 5 mins

Servings – 1

What You Need:

- 1% cottage cheese, ½ cup
- Truvia baking blend, 1 tsp
- Dash of ginger
- Dash of cloves
- Dash of cinnamon
- Canned pumpkin, ½ cup
- Old fashioned oats, ⅓ cup

What You Do:

1. Place the sweetener, spices, pumpkin, and oats in a microwave safe bowl.
2. Cook on high for 90 seconds in the microwave and then stir in the cottagecheese.
3. Allow this to microwave for another 60 seconds.
4. Allow this to stand for a few minutes before eating.

Calories: 205

Fat: 3 g

Protein: 14 g

Carb: 34 g

Baked Tomatoes

Prep: 10 mins

Cook: 50 mins

Servings – 6

What You Need:

- Pine nuts, ¼ cup
- Greek seasoning
- Low-fat parmesan cheese, ¼ cup
- Olive oil spray
- Large tomatoes, 5-6

What You Do:

1. Set your oven to 350 degrees.
2. Slice the tomatoes in half lengthwise and place them cut side up in a pan.Spray the tops of the tomato with olive oil spray.
3. Sprinkle on the pine nuts and cheese and some Greek seasoning.
4. Allow them to bake for 50 minutes.
5. Serving size is a whole tomato.

Calories: 73

Fat: 5 g

Protein: 3 g

Carb: 6 g

Classic Hummus

Prep: 5 mins

Cook: 5 mins

Servings – 12

What You Need:

- Salt, ½ tsp

- Fresh lemon juice, 3 tbs

- Tahini, 1 tbs

- Extra virgin olive oil, 3 tbs

- Rinsed chickpeas, 15 oz

- Smashed garlic clove, 1

What You Do:

1. Place the garlic in a food processor until finely minced. Scrape the sides downand add in the salt, tahini, oil, lemon juice, and chickpeas. Mix this until it becomes completely smooth. Scrape the sides down when necessary.

Calories: 72

Fat: 4.5 g

Protein: 1.5 g

Carb: 7.5 g

Cheesecake Pudding Recipe

Prep: 5 mins

Cook: 0 mins

Servings – 4

What You Need:

- Sugar-free cheesecake pudding, 1 pack
- Fat-free Greek yogurt, 1 cup

What You Do:

1. Place both ingredients in a blender and mix until smooth.

Calories: 20

Fat: 0 g

Protein: 7 g

Carb: 2.7 g

Creamy Cauliflower Puree

Prep: 10 mins

Cook: 0 mins

Servings – 4

What You Need:

- Pepper, ½ tsp

- Extra virgin olive oil, 4 tsp

- Garlic salt, ½ tsp

- Salted butter, 1 tsp

- Low-fat buttermilk, ⅓ cup

- Garlic, 3 cloves

- Large head of cauliflower

What You Do:

2. Break up the cauliflower into small florets and place them in a large microwave bowlalong with the garlic and a quarter cup of water.

3. Microwave for five minutes or until the cauliflower has become tender.

4. With a garlic press, crush the garlic cloves and add them to a food processor. Add inthe cauliflower. Pour in the pepper, garlic salt, butter, two teaspoons of olive oil, and buttermilk.

5. Process everything together until creamy and smooth.

6. Drizzle in the rest of the olive oil and serve.Calories: 113

Fat: 6 g

Protein: 5 g

Carb: 13 g

Tuna Salad

Prep: 10 mins

Cook: 0 mins

Servings – 4

What You Need:

- Powdered eggs, 1 tbs
- Mayonnaise, 1 ½ tbs
- Pickle juice, 1 tbs
- Drained tuna packed in water, 6 oz can

What You Do:

1. Place all of the ingredients into a blender and mix until smooth. Enjoy

.Calories: 138

Fat: 7.4 g

Protein: 12.1 g

Carb: 5.4 g

Overnight Oats

Prep: 3 mins

Cook: 12 hrs

Servings – 4

What You Need:

- Fat-free Greek yogurt, ¾ cup
- Protein powder, 2 tbs
- Semi-skimmed milk, 1 ¼ cup
- Chia seeds, 2 tbs
- Porridge oats, 1 cup

What You Do:

1. Make sure you make the recipe the night before you plan on eating it.

2. Combine the yogurt, protein powder, milk, chia seeds, and oats together in a bowl. Spoon the mixture into four individual servings and cover them. Allow the mixture to sit in the fridge overnight.

3. To serve, stir the mixture again and enjoy. You can also top with seeds, nuts, or fruitsif desired.

Calories: 338

Fat: 10.9 g

Protein: 22.8 g

Carb: 34.7 g

Winter Sunshine Smoothie

Prep: 1 mins

Cook: 0 mins

Servings – 1

What You Need:

- Fresh ginger, ½ inch piece
- Fresh turmeric, ½ inch piece
- Segmented and peeled clementines, 2
- Unsweetened coconut milk, 2 tbs
- Chilled unsweetened coconut water, 1 cup
- Rolled porridge oats, ⅓ cup

What You Do:

1. Add the oats to a blender and pulse until it turns into a finely ground powder.
2. Add in the ginger, turmeric, clementines, coconut milk, and coconut water andpulse until they come together.
3. Pour your smoothie into a glass and enjoy.

Calories: 192

Fat: 2.1 g

Protein: 5.1 g

Carb: 40.8 g

Chocolate Porridge

Prep: 1 mins

Cook: 3 mins

Servings – 1

What You Need:

- Blackberries
- Small square dark unsweetened chocolate
- Low-cal sweetener, 1 tbs
- Chocolate protein powder, 1 tbs
- Porridge oats, 3 tbs
- Skimmed milk, 1 cup

What You Do:

1. Add the chocolate, protein powder, oats, and milk to a jug and mix everythingtogether.
2. Place the container in the microwave and cook for two minutes.
3. Stir everything together again and let it cook for another 20 to 30 seconds.
4. Mix in your sweetener of choice.
5. Spoon into a serving bowl and top with a couple of blackberries and a little bit ofchopped chocolate.

Calories: 328

Fat: 7.2 g

Protein: 23.3 g

Carb: 41.8 g

Mugastrone

Prep: 1 mins

Cook: 5 mins

Servings – 1

What You Need:

- PepperSalt
- Dry vermicelli, .25 oz
- Frozen mixed vegetables, 1 ½ tbs
- Cooked borlotti beans, 1 tbs
- Tomato juice, ⅔ cup

What You Do:

1. Add the tomato sauce into a glass measuring cup and then add in some pepper,salt, noodles, vegetables, and beans. Stir everything together.

2. Place in the microwave and cook for two to three minutes.

3. If you want, you can cook it on the stove. Place everything in a pot and bring itto a boil. Cook for around three to four minutes or until the noodles are cookedthrough.

4. You can top with some parmesan, basil, or pesto if desired.

Calories: 170

Fat: .4 g

Protein: 4.1 g

Carb: 16.8 g

Phase Four Recipes

Steak Fajitas

Prep: 15 mins

Cook: 30 mins

Servings – 4

What You Need:

- Salsa

- Onion that has been sliced into strips

- Green bell pepper that has been sliced into strips

- Dried thyme, ½ tsp

- Mustard powder, ½ tsp

- Black pepper, 1 tsp

- Cumin, 1 tsp

- Dried rosemary, 2 tsp

- Chili powder, 2 tsp

- Natural sweetener, 2 packets

- Paprika, 1 tbs

- Sea salt, 1 tbs

- Lean sirloin steak, 1 pound, cut into strips

What You Do:

1. Place the salt, paprika, sweetener, chili powder, dried rosemary, cumin, pepper, mustard powder, and dried thyme into a bowl and mix well to combine. Take out one teaspoon of this mixture and reserve. Rub the steak slices really well with the spice mixture that you just made. Cover the steak and allow it to marinate until you are ready to

cook it.

2. Place a large skillet on the stove and heat to medium-high. Add the onion and pepper to the skillet along with the spice mixture that you set to the side earlier.You need to cook the onion and peppers until they have softened up and the onions turn translucent. Take off heat and place in a bowl. Cover to keep warm.

3. Into the same skillet, add half the seasoned steak and cook for about two minutesper side or until done to your liking. Place cooked steak onto a clean plate and cover until the rest of the steak gets done.

4. Once all the steak strips are done, add everything back into the skillet and warmeverything up for a few minutes. Spoon onto plates and enjoy.

Calories: 663

Fat: 22.1 g

Protein: 104.7

Carb: 6 g

Pumpkin and Black Bean Soup

Prep: 10 mins

Cook: 35 mins

Servings – 6

What You Need:

- Pumpkin puree, 16 oz
- Cumin, 1 tbs
- Vegetable broth, 2 cups
- Diced tomatoes, 1 cup
- Rinsed black beans, 2 15 oz cans
- Pepper, ½ tsp
- Chili powder, 1 tsp
- Minced garlic, 4 cloves
- Chopped onion, 1 medium
- Olive oil, 2 tbs

What You Do:

1. Place the oil in a large pot on medium heat. Once warmed, add the pepper, chili powder, cumin, garlic, and onions. Cook until they soften.

2. Mix in the pumpkin, broth, tomatoes, and black beans.

3. Allow the mixture to simmer, uncovered, for around 25 minutes, or until the soup has thickened. Stir the mixture occasionally.

4. You can serve as is, or you can puree it with an immersion blender until smooth. Calories: 290

Fat: 6 g

Protein: 15 g

Carb: 46 g

Greek Yogurt Chicken

Prep: 10 mins

Cook: 45 mins

Servings – 4

What You Need:

- Garlic powder, 1 tsp
- Pepper, ½ tsp
- Seasoning salt, 1 ½ tsp
- Parmesan cheese, ½ cup
- Greek yogurt, 1 cup
- Skinless, boneless chicken breasts, 4

What You Do:

1. Start by setting your oven to 375 degrees.
2. Mix together the seasonings, cheese, and Greek yogurt.
3. Lay some tin foil on a baking sheet and spritz it with some nonstick spray.
4. Spread the Greek yogurt mixture over the chicken breasts and lay them on theprepared baking sheet.
5. Slide them into the oven and let them cook for 45 minutes.

Calories: 266

Fat: 4 g

Protein: 46 g

Carb: 3 g

Whopper Veggie Burger

Prep: 5 mins

Cook: 15 mins

Servings – 1

What You Need:

- Onion, 1
- Tomato, 1
- Lettuce
- Mustard, 1 tbs
- Ketchup, 1 tbs
- Light miracle whip, 1 tbs
- While wheat hamburger bun, 1
- Boca burger, 1

What You Do:

1. Following the directions on the package, cook the Boca burger until done.

2. Place the burger on the bun and top it with all of the other toppings andcondiments.

Calories: 260

Fat: 5.5 g

Protein: 18 g

Carb: 40 g

Brown Rice and Black Bean Casserole

Prep: 10 mins

Cook: 1 hr 25 mins

Servings – 8

What You Need:

- Low-fat Swiss cheese, 2 cups
- Shredded carrots, ⅓ cup
- Diced green chilies, 4 oz
- Drained black beans, 15 oz
- Cayenne pepper, ¼ tsp
- Cumin, ½ tsp
- Sliced mushrooms, ½ cup
- Cooked, chopped, skinless, boneless chicken breast, 16 oz
- Sliced zucchini
- Diced onion, ⅓ cup
- Olive oil, 1 tbsp
- Vegetable broth, 1 cup
- Brown rice, ⅓ cup

What You Do:

1. Combine the rice with the vegetable broths and allow it to come to a boil. Turn the heat down and allow the mixture to simmer for 45 minutes, or until the rice iscooked.

2. Set your oven to 350 degrees.

3. Grease a casserole dish with some cooking spray.

4. Add the oil to a skillet and heat to medium. Mix in the onion until tender.

5. Stir in the seasonings, mushrooms, chicken, and zucchini.

6. Stir and cook this mixture until the zucchini has lightly browned and chicken isheated through.

7. In a large bowl, combine a cup of cheese, carrots, chilies, beans, mushrooms,chicken, zucchini, onion, and rice.

8. Pour this mixture into your casserole dish and cover it with the rest of thecheese.

9. Loosely tent some tin foil over the top and bake it for 30 minutes in the oven.

10. Remove the foil and let it continue to bake for ten minutes, or until the cheesehas browned.

Calories: 267

Fat: 6 g

Protein: 31 g

Carb: 22 g

Shrimp Ceviche

Prep: 25 mins

Cook: 20 mins

Servings – 4

What You Need:

- Serrano chili peppers, 2
- Chopped bunch of cilantro
- Small red onion, chopped
- Medium tomatoes, 4
- Lime juice, 1 cup
- Medium raw shrimp, 1 lb

What You Do:

1. Place the lime juice and shrimp in a bowl and toss together. Cover and allow the shrimp to marinade for ten to 15 minutes. The color should change to pink. Don't allow them to marinate for too long; otherwise, the shrimp will become overcooked.

2. Add in the cilantro, chili peppers, tomatoes, and onion.

3. Stir everything together gently.

4. Season with some salt.

5. Serve cold

Calories: 160

Fat: 1 g

Protein: 25 g

Carb: 13 g

Taco Beef

Prep: 15 mins

Cook: 8 hrs

Servings – 6

What You Need:

- Chipotle pepper in adobo sauce, minced, 1
- Minced garlic, 5 cloves
- Chili powder, 2 tsp
- Small white onion, diced, 1
- Chuck tender roast, 2 lb
- Tomato paste, 2 tbs
- Beef broth, low sodium, 1 cup
- Paprika, ½ tsp
- Cumin, 1 tsp
- Olive oil, 2 tsp

What You Do:

1. Place paprika, cumin, and chili powder into a small bowl and mix everythingtogether. Rub this mixture into the chuck roast. Make sure that you cover thechuck roast well.

2. Set a large pan on top of the stove and warm it to medium-high. Add in the oliveoil and let it get hot. Place beef into the skillet and sear for two minutes. Turn theroast and sear every side. Take the beef out of the skillet and put into the bottom of slow cooker.

3. Add the diced onion into the skillet you seared the beef in and cook for threeminutes until onions become soft and translucent. Mix in the garlic, cookinguntil fragrant. Pour the beef broth into the skillet and scrape with a wooden spoon to deglaze the pan.

4. Add the minced chipotle and tomato paste into the skillet and using a whisk, stiruntil everything is combined. Allow the mixture to come up to a boil and then turn the heat down until it simmers. Let it simmer for five minutes, or until it hasthickened. Take off heat and pour over beef in bottom of slow cooker.

5. Place lid on slow cooker and set on low. Cook for eight hours until the beef willshred easily with a fork.

6. When beef is done, take it out of the cooker and shred it up. Mix it back into thejuices so that it is well coated.

7. Use as you would any meat mixture in your favorite Mexican dishes or eat as is.

Calories: 292

Fat: 11.1 g

Protein: 42.3 g

Carb: 4 g

Slow cooker Chicken Enchiladas

Prep: 15 mins

Cook: 4 hrs 45 mins

Servings – 5

What You Need:

- Medium whole grain tortillas, 6 (make sure they are not corn because they tend to fall aparteasily)
- Garlic powder, ½ tsp
- Fat-free sour cream, 8 oz
- Pepper, ½ tsp
- Chili powder, 1 tsp
- Reduced fat shredded cheddar cheese, 1 ½ cups
- Cumin, 1 tsp
- Can of jalapenos, 4 oz
- No sugar added red enchilada sauce, 16 oz
- Skinless chicken breast fillets, 2

What You Do:

1. Start by setting the oven to 350 degrees.

2. Place aluminum foil on a baking dish and lay the chicken in the bottom of thedish.

3. Place the chicken in the oven and cook until it has clear juices when pierced witha fork. This should take about 35 to 45 minutes.

4. If you chicken had skin on it, remove the skin at this point.

5. Shred up the chicken, or you can cut them into bite-sized pieces.

6. Grab a decent-sized bowl and add in the pepper, chili powder, garlic powder, cumin, and chicken. Add in a pinch of salt, or however much your taste buds sayyou need.

7. Toss everything together until the chicken is well coated in the seasonings.

8. To this mixture, add a cup of cheese, a half cup of sour cream, a half cup of enchilada sauce, and jalapeno pepper. Mix everything together so that everything is well distributed.

9. Add a half cup of the chicken mixture onto the center of every tortilla. Make sure that you leave around two inches at the bottom of the tortilla clean and foldthe tortilla over the filling.

10. Continue folding until you have finished all of the enchiladas.

11. Stack all of your enchiladas into your slow cooker. Add some of the enchilada sauce on top of each of the layers of enchiladas as you stack them in.

12. There will typically be two layers of three enchiladas or three layers of twoenchiladas, depending on the size and shape of your slow cooker.

13. Mix the rest of the enchilada sauce with a half a cup of sour cream. Pour this

14. mixture over top of the enchilada.

15. Place the lid on the cooker and allow them to cook for three to four hours onlow, or until everything is hot and bubbly.

16. Cut between the enchiladas and carefully take them out, one enchilada at a time,using a large spatula.

17. Using a spoon, pour the liquid that is left in the slow cooker over yourenchiladas, and sprinkle them with the rest of the cheese.

18. Garnish your enchiladas with shredded lettuce and diced tomatoes.

Calories: 263

Fat: 6.2 g

Protein: 16.3 g

Carb: 34.2 g

Creamy Green Chile Enchilada Soup

Prep: 20 mins

Cook: 7 hrs 50 mins

Servings – 10

What You Need:
- Corn starch, 1 tbs (if needed)
- Pepper
- Garlic powder, 1 tsp
- Salt
- Uncooked instant rice, ¾ cup
- Chili powder, 1 tbs
- Cream cheese, 8 oz
- Frozen corn, 1 cup
- Onion powder, 1 tsp
- Ground cumin, 2 tbs
- Water, ¾ cup
- Diced green chilies, 4 oz
- Green chili enchilada sauce, 2 cans
- Chicken breasts, 24 oz
- Chicken broth, 32 oz
- Optional toppings: sour cream, avocado, and shredded cheese

What You Do:
1. In your slow cooker, combine together the cumin, onion

powder, garlic powder,chili powder, water, green chilies, green enchilada sauce, and broth.

2.   You can adjust any of the amounts of seasonings to your taste.

3.   Snuggle the chicken breasts into the mixture in the slow cooker and cover thecooker with the lid. Set the cooker to cook for seven hours on low.

4.   Once you hit the seven-hour mark, take the chicken out of the cooker and placeit in another dish.

5.   Shred up the chicken and then mix it back into the mixture in the cooker.

6.   Mix in the cream cheese, corn, and instant rice to your soup mixture and put thelid back on the cooker.

7.   Allow the mixture to cook for another 30 minutes.

8.   Stir the soup again; making sure that all of the cream cheese is well distributed and melted. You may have to cook the mixture a bit longer to make sure that thecream cheese does get completely melted.

9.   Now you need to judge the consistency of the soup in your cooker.

10. If you want the soup to be a bit thicker, you can mix in a tablespoon of cornstarch into an eighth of a cup of water and then stir this back into your soup.Keep the lid off and allow the soup to thicken for about ten to 20 minutes.

11. If you see that the soup is already thick enough for your taste, you can skip thisstep.

12. Feel free to use chicken thighs in this recipe if you want a little extra flavor. Theimportant thing to remember is to make sure that you remove as much fat from the thighs as

you can before you start to cook anything.

Calories: 339

Fat: 15 g

Protein: 26.3 g

Carb: 25.5 g

Tilapia Veracruz

Prep: 10 mins

Cook: 20 mins

Servings – 6

What You Need:

- Lime, 1
- Capers, 2 tbs
- Green olives, ¼ cup
- Crushed tomatoes, 2 cups
- Chopped oregano, ½ tsp
- Bay leaves, 2
- Sliced garlic, 3 cloves
- Sliced Anaheim chili, 1
- Sliced onion, 1
- Salt
- Tilapia fillets, 6
- Extra virgin olive oil, 2 tbs

What You Do:

1. Place the oil in a large pan and allow it to heat on medium-high.
2. Season both sides of the fish fillets with some pepper and salt. Make sure youlightly press the seasoning in with your fingers.

3. Place the fish into your hot skillet and allow them to cook until they are goldenbrown on the bottom. This should take three to four minutes.

4. Flip the fish carefully and allow it to cook for another two minutes.

5. Take the fish out and set it on a plate while you cook everything else.

6. Add the chili and the onion to your skillet and sauté it for two to three minutes oruntil the onions have softened.

7. Mix in the garlic and cook it for 30 seconds.

8. Mix in the capers, green olives, crushed tomatoes, oregano, and bay leaves intothe mixtures. Allow this to come to a simmer and cook until it has thickened slightly, around five minutes.

9. Place the fish back into your pan and let it simmer for three to four minutesmore, or until the fish has cooked all the way through.

10. The fish should be opaque and should easily flake once cooked through. Takethe bay leaves out of the mixture. Serve with a lime wedge.

11. Oven Method:

12. Set your oven at 350 degrees.

13. Add the oil to the bottom of a nine by 13-inch baking dish.

14. Place the fillets in the bottom of the pan. Frozen fillets work best for thiscooking method.

15. Place all the remaining ingredients on top of the fish, minus the lime wedge.

16. Allow this mixture to cook until the fish flakes easily with a

fork. This shouldtake between 20 to 30 minutes.

Calories: 543

Fat: 19.4 g

Protein: 85.1 g

Carb: 6.5 g

Taco Pie

Prep: 10 mins

Cook: 30 mins

Servings – 8

What You Need:

- 2% cheddar cheese, ⅔ cup, shredded
- Pepper
- Salt
- Large eggs, 6
- Water, ¾ cup
- Taco seasoning packet 93% lean ground beef, 1 lb
- Toppings of choice

What You Do:

1. Start by setting your oven to 350 degrees.

2. Place your pan on a stove and allow it to heat up to medium-high. Once theskillet has heated up, add the ground beef and cook for about five minutes, breaking it apart as it cooks.

3. Cook it until it is completely browned and no longer pink. If there is any fat, drain it off. Mix in the taco seasoning and water. Mix everything together andallow it to simmer until the water is absorbed (about five minutes.)

4. Spray a nine-inch pie pan with nonstick spray. Place the beef mixture into the piepan evenly.

5. Crack the eggs in a bowl and whisk in some pepper and salt. Whisk until wellcombined. Pour eggs over beef mixture and tilt the pie pan to make sure eggscover the beef mixture completely.

6. Sprinkle cheese on top. Place it in the oven and cook for about 25 minutes. After25 minutes, check pie and see if the eggs are set. If not, cook an additional five minutes.

7. When done, take it out of the oven and allow it to cool. Slice evenly and servewith toppings of choice.

Calories: 147

Fat: 7.3 g

Protein: 18.2 g

Carb: .9 g

Slow Cooker Carnitas "Nachos"

Prep: 10 mins

Cook: 6 hrs 10 mins

Servings – 6

What You Need:

- Mini sweet peppers, 1 bag
- Salt, ¾ tsp
- Cumin, 1 tbs
- Chicken broth, 10 ounce can
- Chipotle peppers in adobo sauce, 7 ounce can
- Minced garlic, 4 cloves
- Lean pork shoulder, 2 pounds
- Toppings:
- Cilantro, chopped, 2 tbs
- 2% shredded cheddar cheese, ½ cup

What You Do:

1. If you don't like cleaning a slow cooker, use a slow cooker liner or spray it wellwith some nonstick spray.

2. Pour the chicken broth, chipotle peppers along with the sauce, salt, cumin, and garlic in the bottom of your slow cooker. Stir well to mix. Add the pork shoulderand turn to coat all sides.

3. Place the pork shoulder in your slow cooker and sit the lid on top. Turn the slowcooker onto low and set for six hours.

When done, take the pork out and shred it.Add it back to the sauce and mix together to coat with the sauce.

4. Warm your oven to 350 degrees. Slice the bell peppers in half and remove the seeds. Place evenly onto a baking pan. Spread shredded pork onto bell peppersevenly. Add on the cheese. Place in preheated oven and bake for ten minutes.

5. Once the cheese is melted, take it out of the oven and top with toppings ofchoice. Enjoy.

Calories: 561

Fat: 32.1 g

Protein: 61.4 g

Carb: 3.1 g

Chipotle Steak Salad

Prep: 10 mins

Cook: 10 mins

Servings – 4

What You Need:

- Reduced fat cheddar cheese, ½ cup, shredded
- Chopped cilantro, 1 tbs
- Sliced avocado, ½
- Diced and seeded tomato, 1
- Washed and torn, romaine lettuce, 1 head
- Taco seasoning packet, ½
- Lean steaks, 4 Toppings of choice

What You Do:

1. Begin by heating a grill or grill pan to medium. Rub the taco seasoning into themeat, making sure it is well coated. Set this aside to let it marinade.

2. Once your grill is hot, place steaks on the grill and cook for five minutes per sideuntil it reaches your desired doneness.

3. Take off the grill and place on cutting board. Allow the meat to rest for aboutfour minutes.

4. While steaks are cooking, wash and tear lettuce. Divide out among four plates.

5. Slice the steaks across the grain and add on top of the lettuce. Add avocado, tomato, and cilantro. Sprinkle with

cheese. Use salsa as the salad dressing if youwould like to. Enjoy.

Calories: 360

Fat: 25.6 g

Protein: 23.9 g

Carb: 9.5 g

Chile Relleno Casserole

Prep: 10 mins

Cook: 25 mins

Servings – 4

What You Need:

- For topping:
- Salt
- Mexican blend cheese, shredded, 1 cup
- Diced green chilies, 7 ounces
- Flour, 2 tbs Milk, ¾ cup
- Eggs, 2
- For beef mixture:
- Taco seasoning, 1 tbs
- Ground beef, 1 pound

What You Do:

1. The first thing you need to do is preheat your oven to 350 degrees.

2. Place a skillet on the stove and heat to medium-high. Add in the ground beef andallow it to cook until it is completely browned.

3. Make sure you break the beef into smaller pieces as it cooks up. If the beefaccumulates any grease as it cooks, make sure to drain it all off. Add taco seasoning and stir well to combine.

4. Use cooking spray and spray an eight by eight-inch pan. Place seasoned groundbeef in bottom of the pan.

5. Crack the eggs into a bowl and add flour and milk. Whisk until there aren't anylumps left in the mixture. Mix in the green chilies and the cheese. Mix everything together.

6. Pour the eggs over the beef and put in the preheated oven. Bake for 20 minutesuntil top is golden brown.

Calories: 524

Fat: 24 g

Protein: 63.7 g

Carb: 8.5 g

Steak and Mushroom Fajita Sandwiches

Prep: 10 mins

Cook: 40 mins

Servings – 4

What You Need:

- Fat-free sour cream, ¼ cup

- Romaine lettuce leaves, torn, 4

- Whole wheat tortillas, 4

- Salt Pepper

- Dried oregano, 2 tsp

- Beef sirloin tip steak, cut into strips, 1 pound

- Medium red bell pepper, cut into strips

- 1 Minced garlic, 2 cloves

- Medium red onion, sliced into strips, 1O

- olive oil, 1 tbs plus 2 tsp

What You Do:

1. Set your oven to 350 degrees.

2. Set a large pan on top of the stove and warm it to medium-high. Add onetablespoon of olive oil and allow to warm up.

3. Put mushroom in the skillet and cook for about six minutes until softened. Add garlic, bell peppers, and onions. Continue to cook until the peppers and onionsare softened. This should take about four minutes.

4. Add in beef and lower the heat to medium. Cook for about ten minutes until beef is no longer pink. Sprinkle with oregano, pepper, and salt. Stir everything together really well to make sure that all of the seasonings are evenly distributed.

5. Turn the heat down and let it simmer, covered. Let the mixture simmer aboutfive minutes. Drain the mixture if you find that it has accumulated any fat.

6. Stack the tortillas together and wrap them in aluminum foil. Put them on the baking sheet and bake for 15 minutes. Take tortillas out of the oven and carefullyunwrap.

7. Divide the meat mixture among the four tortillas and top with lettuce and sourcream if desired. Enjoy.

Calories: 488

Fat: 20.7 g

Protein: 40.6 g

Carb: 32.9 g

Chili Lime Jalapeno Turkey Burgers

Prep: 10 mins

Cook: 15 mins

Servings – 8

What You Need:

- Egg white, 1

- Sea salt

- Lime juice, 2 tbs

- Diced green onions, 2 tbs

- Seeded and chopped jalapeno, 1 small

- 93% lean ground turkey, 1 pound

- Toppings of choice:

- Spinach Tomato slices

What You Do:

1. Place a nonstick grill pan on the stove and heat to medium-high.

2. While the grill pan is heating, chop the green onions and jalapeno very finely.

3. Place the egg white, salt, lime juice, green onion, garlic, jalapeno, and turkeyinto a bowl.

4. Using your hands, mix well until everything is combined. Divide out into eightportions and form into eight patties.

5. Cook the burgers in batches. Place the burgers onto the preheated grill pan. Cookthe burgers for one minute to sear one side.

6. Cover with a large lid in order to keep the steam in and keep the burger moist.Only do this after the first side has been seared. Cook under the lid for four minutes. Turn burger over and repeat on the other side.

7. Check the internal temperature of the burger. Make sure the internal temperaturehas reached at least 165 degrees.

8. Once cooked thoroughly, place on plates and add your toppings of choice. Serveand enjoy.

Calories: 185

Fat: 8.2 g

Protein: 22.8 g

Carb: 2.3 g

Cilantro Lime Chicken with Tomato Relish

Prep: 5 mins

Cook: 20 mins

Servings – 4

What You Need:

- Pepper

- Salt

- Cumin, 2 tsp

- Skinless, boneless chicken breast tenders, 1 pound

- Halved cherry tomatoes, 10

- Lime juice, ½ of a lime

- Chopped cilantro, 2 tbs

- Chopped green onions, 3

What You Do:

1. Put the tomatoes, lime juice, cilantro, and green onions into a medium bowl. Cover the bowl and place it in the refrigerator until ready to use. This allows the flavors to marinate.

2. Place the chicken on a plate and season all sides with pepper, salt, and cumin.

3. Set the skillet over medium-high. You might have to cook these in batches. Placesome chicken into the heated skillet and cook five minutes on each side. Make sure that you

check the chicken's internal temperature and make sure that it comes up to 165 degrees. Remove from skillet and place on a plate. Make sure tokeep it warm.

4. Continue cooking chicken until all tenders have been cooked to an internaltemperature of 165 degrees.

5. When all the chicken tenders are done, place on a plate and top with the tomato-lime relish. Serve and enjoy.

Calories: 302

Fat: 8.3 g

Protein: 51.2 g

Carb: 4.5 g

Turkey Skillet with Salsa and Eggs

Prep: 5 mins

Cook: 15 mins

Servings – 4

What You Need:

- Pepper

- Salt

- Cumin, ½ teaspoon

- Large eggs, 4

- Salsa, 16-ounce jar

- 93% lean ground turkey, 1 pound

What You Do:

1. Lay a pan over medium-high heat. Add in the ground turkey and allow it to cookuntil it is completely browned.

2. As the turkey is cooking, make sure that you break it into smaller pieces. If itaccumulates any fat, make sure that you drain it off before continuing.

3. Mix in the salsa and cumin and mix everything together. Allow it to come to aboil. Place the heat on low and let it simmer. Make four wells in the mixture tohold each egg.

4. Crack one egg into each well. Sprinkle tops of eggs with pepper and salt. Coverskillet with a lid. Continue to simmer for about eight minutes until eggs have setup to the desired doneness.

5. Take off heat and cool for a bit. Serve and enjoy.

Calories: 430

Fat: 21.1 g

Protein: 49.3 g

Carb: 4.6 g

Chicken Chili with Jalapeno and Cheddar

Prep: 10 mins

Cook: 40 mins

Servings – 4

- **What You Need:**
- Diced carrots, 1 cup
- Cumin, 1 tbs
- Shredded pepper jack cheese, ½ cup
- Low fat cream cheese, ¼ cup
- Chicken broth, ½ cup
- Oregano, 1 tsp
- Chili powder, 1 tbs
- Diced jarred jalapeno slices, ⅓ cup
- Skinless, boneless chicken breast, 1 pound

What You Do:

1. Spray a Dutch oven with cooking spray. Place the Dutch oven over medium-highheat.

2. Add in the diced chicken along with the diced jalapenos. Cook until chickenturns opaque.

3. Add oregano, chili powder, and cumin to the chicken and jalapenos. Stir everything together so that it is well combined.

4. Mix in the carrots and chicken broth. Stir to combine. Bring to a boil. Onceboiling, turn heat down to low and cover.

5. Allow this mixture to simmer for 20 minutes until the carrots are soft.

6. Add in pepper jack and cream cheese. Stir until mixed well and cheese is melted.Allow it to simmer for five minutes more.

7. Divide evenly into bowls.

8. Serve and enjoy.

Calories: 450

Fat: 18.2 g

Protein: 61.7 g

Carb: 7.9 g

Grilled Chicken with Pico de Gallo

Prep: 15 mins

Cook: 15 mins

Servings – 4

What You Need:

- Minced garlic, 1 clove
- Diced jalapeno pepper, 1
- Diced onion, ½ cup
- Seeded and diced Roma tomatoes, 4
- Pepper
- Salt Limes, 2
- Cilantro, 1 bunch
- Skinless, boneless chicken breast tenders, 1 pound

What You Do:

1. Place a nonstick grill pan on top of stove and heat to medium-high or preheat aregular grill.

2. Place one teaspoon of salt, juice of one lime, and one cup of chopped cilantro ina shallow dish. Stir to combine. Mix in the chicken and stir everything together.Set aside and let marinate for at least 15 minutes.

3. While the chicken is marinating, dice up the garlic, onions, a handful of cilantro, jalapeno, and tomatoes. Mix well to combine all flavors.

4. Add in some pepper and salt. Add in the juice of the other

lime and mix again tocombine everything. Set aside until ready to serve.

5. Take the chicken out of the marinade and put it on your preheated grill.

6. Let this cook for around five minutes on both sides until it reaches 165 degrees.When cooked through, place chicken tenders on plate and top with the Pico de Gallo mixture.

Calories: 337

Fat: 8.3 g

Protein: 53.3 g

Carb: 11 g

Turkey Taco Meatballs

Prep: 10 mins

Cook: 15 mins

Servings – 6

What You Need:

- Chopped cilantro
- 2% cheddar cheese, 12 cubes
- Taco seasoning, 1 packet
- Chopped garlic, 1 tbs
- Eggs, 2
- Chopped green onions, ½ cup
- 93% lean ground turkey, 1 pound

What You Do:

1. Preheat oven to 425 degrees.
2. Place the eggs in a bowl and beat them slightly. Add garlic, green onions, tacoseasoning, and turkey.
3. Using your hands, mix until everything is combined well. Divide the turkeymixture into six even balls.
4. Take one cheese cube and press into the center of a turkey ball. Make sure thecheese is completely encased within the turkey.
5. Place some tin foil on a baking sheet and spray with nonstick spray. Put intopreheated oven and cook for ten minutes, or until golden.

6. Sprinkle with chopped cilantro and shredded cheese.

7. Serve and enjoy

.Calories: 358

Fat: 19.7 g

Protein: 36.2 g

Carb: 3.6 g

Seven Layer Mexican Salad

Prep: 20 mins

Cooke: 30 mins

Servings – 8

What You Need:

Dressing:

- Garlic salt, ¼ tsp
- Cumin, ½ tsp
- Olive oil, 1 tbs
- Lime juice, 2 limes
- Jalapeno, ½
- Cilantro, ¼ cup
- Avocado

Salad:

- Chopped green onions, 2
- Low-fat shredded cheddar cheese, 1 cup
- Diced bell pepper
- Can of drained corn
- Can of drained and rinsed black beans
- Diced tomatoes, 1 cup
- Chopped romaine lettuce, 2 cups
- Box of Jiffy cornbread

What You Do:

1. Dressing:

2. Place all of the ingredients for the dressing in your blender and pulse them untilthe cilantro is well blended into the avocado and lime juice.

3. Salad:

4. First, prepare the cornbread according to the directions on the box.

5. Once it has cooked through, set it aside and allow it to cool completely.

6. Once it is cooled, cut the cornbread in half and then break half of it up into littlecrumbs.

7. Put the crumbled cornbread into the bottom of your dish.

8. Using a trifle dish is best because you will be able to see all of the beautifullayers. You can use any bowl that you want if you don't have a trifle dish.

9. Place half of the romaine lettuce on top of the crumbled cornbread. Make sureyou evenly spread it across. This is your second layer.

10. Top the lettuce with half of the black beans, making sure that they are evenlydistributed.

11. Add half of the corn evenly on top of the beans.

12. Top the corn with half of the chopped bell peppers.

13. Add half of the tomatoes on top of the bell peppers, making sure that they areevenly distributed.

14. Sprinkle half of the cheddar cheese on top of the tomatoes.

15. Now drizzle on half of the salad dressing that you made

earlier.

16. Repeat this process starting with the lettuce through the dressing.

17. To finish the recipe, top everything with the green onions and enjoy.

18. You can reserve the rest of the cornbread for another meal, or you can makeanother salad. The choice is yours.

Calories: 148

Fat: 8.4 g

Protein: 4 g

Carb: 16.8 g

Almond Chicken

Prep: 5 mins

Cook: 20 mins

Servings – 2

What You Need:
- An onion that has been chopped
- Fat-free natural yogurt, 5 ounces
- Ground almonds, 2 tbs
- Skinless, boneless chicken breasts that have been cut into strips, 2
- Black pepper, 1 tsp
- Curry powder, 1 tsp
- Garlic clove, crushed
- Low-fat cooking spray
- Salt, 1 tsp
- Cilantro, chopped for garnish

What You Do:
1. Use the cooking spray and spray a large frying pan generously. Turn the burner on and heat the pan. Once heated, add garlic, curry powder, and onion. Allow this to cook for five minutes.

2. Mix in the chicken to onion mixture and cook for about six minutes until it iscooked through and slightly browned.

3. Lower the heat down to low and mix in the ground almonds. Stir well tocombine everything.

4. Take the pan off of the burner and sprinkle with pepper and salt. Add yogurt andstir well to combine.

5. Sprinkle with cilantro and serve warm

Calories: 302

Fat: 10.4 g

Protein: 36.9 g

Carb: 15.2 g

Autumn Coleslaw

Prep: 5 mins

Cook: 15 mins

Servings – 6

What You Need:

- Flat leaf parsley, chopped, 3 tbs
- Mixed nuts, 2 ounces (chop them if they are large)
- Black pepper
- Salt
- Wholegrain mustard, ½ tsp
- Extra light mayonnaise, 4 tbs
- Fat-free Greek yogurt, 4 tbs
- Lemon, 1 juiced
- Small apples, cored and sliced thin, 2
- A red onion that has been chopped
- Celery, 2 stalks (that have been chopped)
- Red cabbage, shredded, 4 ounces
- White cabbage, shredded, 4 ounces

What You Do:

1. Put the onion, celery, red cabbage, and white cabbage into a large bowl.

2. Add the apples to a bowl and toss them with the lemon juice. Toss to coatwell. Add to the cabbage mixture. Toss to

combine.

3. Add the mustard, mayonnaise, yogurt, pepper, and salt to a different bowl andmix well to combine everything.

4. Pour dressing over the cabbage and apples. Add parsley and nuts. Toss well tocombine all ingredients together.

5. Cover and refrigerate until you are ready to use them. You can even storethem for up to four days.

Calories: 112

Fat: 5.5 g

Protein: 4.9 g

Carb: 10.7 g

Roasted Salmon

Prep: 10 mins

Cook: 14 mins

Servings – 1

What You Need:

- Lemon, 1
- Black pepper
- Salt
- Low-fat cooking spray
- Thin asparagus spears, 3 or 4 Cherry
- tomatoes, 6 cut in half
- Red onion, half of one that has been sliced
- Small salmon fillet
- Spinach leaves, one handful
- Dill for garnish

What You Do:

1. Preheat your oven to 400 degrees.

2. On a cookie sheet, place a large piece of parchment paper or aluminum foil.Place down the handful of spinach leaves. On top of the spinach, place the salmon skin side up.

3. On top of the salmon, place the asparagus, tomatoes, and onion.

4. Give everything a good spray with the cooking spray.

Sprinkle with pepperand salt.

5. Slice the lemon in half and slice one of the halves into slices. Squeeze onehalf of the lemon over the salmon. Place the slices of lemon on top of the salmon.

6. Slide this into the oven for 10 to 14 minutes. It will depend on how thick yoursalmon is as to the cooking time. If you like your vegetables softer, cook them for ten minutes before adding the salmon. Then cook for another ten to 14 minutes.

7. When cooked through, place on a plate and garnish with fresh dill.

Calories: 310

Fat: 15.9 g

Protein: 30.3 g

Carb: 11.3 g

Steak and Potato Skewers

Prep: 15 mins

Cook: 30 mins

Servings – 4

What You Need:

Dressing:

- Water, 4 tbs

- Sugar-free syrup or maple syrup, 1 tbs

- Lemon juice, 2 tbs

- Tahini, 4 tbs

Skewers:

- Black pepper

- Salt

- Low-fat cooking spray

- Cherry tomatoes, 4

- A red onion that has been peeled and cut into wedges Mushrooms

- Multi-colored peppers, 3

- Steak, 1.5 pounds that have been cut into cubes New potatoes, 8 ounces

What You Do:

1. Pour some water into a pot and add salt. Place on a burner and bring to a boil.Wash the potatoes. Cut each one into

quarters or halves depending on their size. Put into the pot of boiling water and cook for eight minutes until tender. Removefrom heat and drain.

2. Put the tomatoes, onions, mushrooms, peppers, and steak into a bowl and spray generously with cooking spray. Sprinkle with pepper and salt. Mix well tocombine.

3. Take the ingredients and alternate them onto four different skewers.

4. Cook them either on an inside or outside grill for ten minutes. Turn themfrequently to ensure even cooking.

5. While skewers are cooking, make the dressing. Place all ingredients for the dressing into a bowl and whisk until incorporated and smooth.

6. When skewers are cooked through, take off grill and place onto serving plates. Drizzle with some of the dressing. Place remaining dressing into a smallbowl for dipping.

Calories: 425

Fat: 16.8 g

Protein: 44.5 g

Carb: 24.7 g

Easy Pork Stir–Fry

Prep: 25 mins

Cook: 10 mins

Servings – 2

What You Need:

- Straight to wok ribbon rice noodles, 5 ounces

- Garlic paste, 1 tsp

- Ginger paste, 1 tsp

- Low-fat cooking spray

- Frozen stir-fry vegetable medley, 7 ounces

- Hoisin sauce, 2 tbs

- Pork, 8 ounces diced

What You Do:

1. Put the pork in a bowl and pour in the hoisin sauce. Mix well to coat and letmarinate for 20 minutes.

2. Take the peppers out of the vegetable medley and slice them thinly. Chop any of the remaining vegetables into smaller pieces if needed.

3. Spray a wok with nonstick spray generously. Put on the burner and heat up. Add garlic and ginger paste and half of the peppers. Cook for one minute. Placethe pork in with the marinade and let it cook for four minutes. Take out of the wok with a slotted spoon and place it to the side.

4. Respray the wok if needed and add in the vegetables and cook for anadditional two minutes.

5. Add the noodles to the wok along with one to two tablespoons of water. Cover and let cook for another two minutes until it reaches the desired doneness.

6. Place the pork back into the wok and toss well to combine.

7. Divide evenly into bowls and top with reserved peppers if you want.

Calories: 315

Fat: 4.3 g

Protein: 30.5 g

Carb: 36.1 g

Ricotta and Spinach Frittata

Prep: 5 mins

Cook: 25 mins

Servings – 3

What You Need:

- Black pepper,Salt
- Skim milk, 3 tbs
- Ricotta, 4 ounces
- Medium eggs, 4 beaten slightly
- An onion that has been sliced thin
- Low-fat cooking spray
- Spinach leaves, 8 ounces
- Small potatoes, 5 ounces, sliced

What You Do:

1. Heat your broiler.

2. Pour water into a pot and generously salt. Allow it to come to a boil. Mix in the potatoes and cook them for around eight minutes until they are tender. Drain.

3. Put the spinach into a large bowl and cover. Place in microwave and cook at full power for two to three minutes until wilted. Squeeze out all the excess liquidand give it a rough chop.

4. Spritz a frying pan with nonstick spray. Put on the burner and heat up. Mix in the onion and let it cook for four

minutes. Add in potatoes and stir well.

5. Add eggs, spinach, milk, ricotta, pepper, and salt to a bowl. Beat well. Pour into the hot pan. Cook gently for four minutes.

6. Carefully put the pan under the broiler for four minutes until it is completelyset and golden brown. Let cool slightly and carefully slide out of the pan. Cut into wedges and serve warm. Have a salad on the side if desired.

Calories: 240

Fat: 11.8 g

Protein: 17 g

Carb: 15.8 g

Puy and Tomato Lentils

Prep: 5 mins

Cook: 15 mins

Servings – 4

What You Need:

- A fat-free dressing of choice, 3 tbs
- Fresh dill, chopped, 2 tbs
- Large tomatoes, 11 ounces
- Gherkin that has been finely chopped
- Baby spinach, 4 ounces
- Cooked Puy lentils, 8 ounces
- Black pepper
- Salt
- White wine vinegar, 1 tbs
- A red onion that has been finely sliced

What You Do:

1. Put the onion in a small bowl. Mix in the salt and white wine vinegar. Toss tocoat and set aside.

2. Place the onions, gherkin, spinach, radishes, and lentils along with a sprinkleof pepper and salt in a bowl and mix everything together.

3. Slice the tomatoes in half and then into individual thick slices. Gently stir intothe lentil mixture until well combined. Add some dill and the dressing. Mix again to coat.

4. Divide evenly onto four plates. Sprinkle with dill and serve.

Calories: 130

Fat: 1.5 g

Protein: 7.6 g

Carb: 19.2 g

Chicken Chili

Prep: 15 mins

Cook: 30 mins

Servings – 6

What You Need:

- Black pepper

- Salt

- Chipotle paste, 2 tsp

- Chicken broth, 2 cups

- Kidney beans, 14-ounce can that has been drained and rinsed

- Red bell pepper, 2 that have been seeded and chopped

- Red split lentils, ½ cup

- Chopped tomatoes, 14 ounces

- Chicken breast fillets, 1.5 pounds

- Ginger root (roughly chopped, then grated), 2 tsp

- One large onion that has been chopped Low-fat cooking spray

- Chopped cilantro to garnish

- Regular or cauliflower rice to serve with

What You Do:

1. Spray a skillet with some nonstick spray. Turn on the burner and heat up. Addin the onion, chicken, and ginger and cook

for about five minutes until chicken is golden brown and cooked through.

2. Add in the tomatoes, pepper, salt, chipotle paste, chicken stock, peppers, and lentils. Stir well and allow to boil. Cover the pot and lower to a simmer. Cook for 25 minutes until pepper and lentils are tender.

3. Divide evenly into bowls and serve. Sprinkle with chopped cilantro. Serve over cauliflower or regular rice if desired.

Calories: 323

Fat: 2.8 g

Protein: 43.4 g

Carb: 35.6 g

Stuffed Romano Peppers

Prep: 10 mins

Cook: 25 mins

Servings – 4

- **What You Need:**

- Fresh parsley, chopped, 2 tbs

- Lemon juice, 1 tbs

- Ready cooked lentils, 8 ounces

- Sun-dried tomatoes, 4 cut into pieces

- Fresh thyme, chopped, 1 tsp

- Garlic cloves, 2 crushed

- Leek that has been finely sliced

- Black pepper

- Salt

- Low-fat cooking spray

- Mixed color peppers, 7 ounces

What You Do:

1. Preheat your oven to 400 degrees.

2. Slice the peppers lengthwise through the stalk. Take out the ribs and seeds and spray all over with cooking spray. Put in an oven proof casserole dish andsprinkle with pepper and salt. Put in oven and bake for 20 minutes.

3. While peppers are baking, coat a skillet with nonstick spray.

Turn on the burner and heat up the pan. Once heated, mix in the thyme, garlic, and leek andlet this cook for another ten minutes, or until soft.

4. Add in the lentils and sun-dried tomatoes and cook for an additional fiveminutes.

5. Add in the parsley and lemon juice and mix well.

6. When the peppers have cooked for 20 minutes, carefully remove them from the oven. Carefully spoon this mixture into the peppers. Place back into the ovenfor five minutes.

7. These can be eaten cold, warm, or hot with a green salad. If you want or need higher protein, you can top with parmesan, goat's cheese, or crumbled feta before placing back into the oven for the last few minutes of cooking.

Calories: 165

Fat: 5.7 g

Protein: 7 g

Carb: 19.1 g

Weetabix Fruitcake

Prep: 5 mins

Cook: 1 hr 15 mins

Servings −16

What You Need:

- Semi-skimmed milk, 1 ¼ cups

- Egg

- Splenda, 1 cup

- Pumpkin spice, 1 tsp

- Weetabix, crushed, 2

- Mixed dried fruit, 1 ⅓ cups

- Baking powder, 3 tsp

- All-purpose flour, 3 cups

- Low-fat cooking spray

What You Do:

1. Preheat your oven to 350 degrees.

2. Coat an eight by four-inch loaf pan with nonstick spray and line withparchment paper.

3. Add the Splenda, pumpkin spice, Weetabix, dried fruit, and flour. Mix well.

4. Gently beat the egg and add milk. Stir together. Mix in the dry ingredients and gently fold until everything is mixed well.

5. Spoon into loaf pan and level the surface. Bake for about one hour and 15minutes. Let cool on a wire rack

6.   Slice and serve.

Calories: 124

Fat: .9 g

Protein: 3.4 g

Carb: 26 g

Pink Lady Cornmeal Cake

Prep: 15 mins

Cook: 1 hr 10 mins

Servings – 12

What You Need:

- Juice and zest of one lemon

- Baking powder, 1 tsp

- Ground almonds, 2 cups

- Salt

- Cornmeal, 1 cup

- Vanilla, 1 tsp

- Eggs, 3 large beaten

- Splenda, ¾ cup

- Butter, ⅔ cup

- Pink lady apple, cored, peeled, and chopped, 1

Topping:

- Pink lady apple, cored and sliced thin, 1

- Confectioner's sugar, ¼ heaped cup

- Zest and juice of one lemon

- Crème fraîche to top

What You Do:

1. Grease and line an eight-inch round cakepan.

2. Place the chopped apple in a little bit of water for about six

minutes until forktender. Take off heat and drain. Let this cool.

3. Beat the sugar and butter together until creamy and light. Slowly mix in the eggs and beat until smooth. Mix in the baking powder, ground almonds, salt, cornmeal, and vanilla. Fold until well combined. Add in the cooled apple, lemon juice, and zest. Stir until well combined.

4. Carefully spoon the batter into your pan and smooth out the top. Slide into theoven for 45 minutes until golden brown and firm.

5. Carefully remove from oven and let it cool for around 20 minutes. Carefullyturn the cake out onto a wire rack so that it can cool entirely.

6. While cake is cooling, make the topping. Add confectioner's sugar, four tablespoons of water, and lemon zest into a pot. Allow it to boil. Place in the sliced apples and allow it to simmer for five minutes. Spoon over the cake andlet cool.

7. Slice into 12 even portions and serve with crème fraiche.

Calories: 253

Fat: 16.2 g

Protein: 7.7 g

Carb: 21.3 g

Chicken Curry

Prep: 15 mins

Cook: 45 mins

Servings – 4

What You Need:

- Cornmeal, 2 tbs
- Cilantro, chopped, 2 tbs
- Chicken stock, ¾ cup
- Light coconut milk, 14 ounces
- Sweet potato, 7 ounces peeled and chopped
- Granny Smith apple that has been peeled, cored, and chopped, 1
- Chicken breast, skinless, boneless, 1 pound, cut into cubes
- Cinnamon stick
- Cardamom pods, 6, crushed
- Ground cumin, 1 tsp
- Turmeric, 1 tsp
- Red chili that has been seeded and chopped, 1
- Garlic cloves, 2 crushed
- One large onion that has been chopped
- Low-fat cooking spray

What You Do:

1. Warm up the skillet on the burner and thenadd the onion

and garlic, cooking until soft. This should take about five minutes. Place in the cinnamon stick, cardamom pods, cumin, turmeric, and chili and cook for an additional two minutes.

2. Place chicken into skillet and cook for three minutes. Stir to combine everything. Add cilantro, chicken stock, coconut milk, sweet potato, and apple.Stir well again. Partially cover the skillet and turn the heat down to a simmer. Let this cook for 35 minutes. Add water as needed.

3. Mix the cornmeal with a small amount of water. Mix together. Add to chickenmixture. Stir well until mixture is slightly thickened.

4. Serve hot over rice if desired.

Calories: 352

Fat: 13.3 g

Protein: 34.1 g

Carb: 24.7 g

Pacific Cod with Fajita Vegetables (Dairy-Free)

Prep: 5 mins

Cook: 15 mins

Servings – 4

What You Need:

- Pepper
- Salt
- Large julienned carrot, 1
- Sliced yellow bell pepper, 2
- Sliced red bell pepper, 2
- Low-fat nonstick spray Scallions, 6
- Juice and zest of a lime
- Wild Alaskan Pacific cod, 4, 6-ounce fillets

What You Do:

1. Heat up your grill or broiler.

2. Place some aluminum foil over the grill rack and place the cod fillets on top.

3. Top the fillets with the lime juice, zest, and some slices of the scallions.

4. Allow them to grill or broil for six to eight minutes, or until it is cooked all the waythrough. The fish will turn opaque and will easily flake once it is cooked through.

5. As the fish cooks, spray a large skillet with some low-fat nonstick spray and allow itto heat up for a few moments on high.

6. Add in the bell peppers, the rest of the scallions, and carrot.

7. Allow them to cook, stirring often, for three to five minutes.

8. Divide your cooked veggies between four different plates and top each of them with acod fillet.

9. Season the top of the fish with some pepper and salt to taste.Calories: 53

Fat: .4 g

Protein: 2.3 g

Carb: 12.8 g

Salmon with Summer Salsa (Dairy–Free)

Prep: 35 mins

Cook: 20 mins

Servings – 4

What You Need:

- Lime wedges

- Chopped cilantro, ¼ cup

- Pepper

- Balsamic vinegar, 1 tbs

- Salt

- Minced red onion, ¼ cup

- Cooked corn kernels, ½ cup

- Olive oil, 1 tsp

- Crushed garlic clove

- Chopped avocado, ½ an avocado

- Chopped tomato, 1 cup

- Skinless salmon, 4, 4-ounce fillets

What You Do:

1. Set your oven to 325 degrees.

2. Stir all of the ingredients together, except for the lime and salmon.

3. Allow the mixture to refrigerate for around 30 minutes so that all of the flavors canmeld together.

4. Place the salmon in your preheated oven and let it cook for 15 to 20 minutes, or untilit has cooked all the way through. The salmon should flake easily and should be opaquewhen it is fully cooked.

5. Serve the cooked salmon topped with the salsa and lime wedge. A great summer option is to allow the salmon to cool off completely after it has cooked. Serving coolsalmon with the chilled salsa is delicious.

Calories: 160

Fat: 9.5 g

Protein: 2 g

Carb: 8 g

Cilantro Lime Cauliflower Rice

Prep: 1 mins

Cook: 5 mins

Servings – 4

What You Need:

- Chopped cilantro, 1 ½ tbs
- Sea salt, ¼ tsp
- Fresh lime juice, 1 tbs
- Frozen riced cauliflower, 10 oz

What You Do:

1. Follow the directions on the package of riced cauliflower to cook it.
2. As the cauliflower is cooking, chop up your cilantro.
3. Take the cauliflower out of the microwave and open the bag to allow all of the steamto release. Make sure that you don't get burned.
4. Pour the cooked cauliflower into a bowl and add in the salt, cilantro, and lime juice.Stir everything together to combine all of the flavors.

Calories: 9

Fat: 0 g

Protein: .5 g

Carb: 1.7 g

Sweet Pepper Poppers

Prep: 5 mins

Cook: 15 mins

Servings – 6

What You Need:

- Salsa, for serving
- 2% shredded cheese, ½ cup
- Chopped cilantro, 2 tbs
- Taco seasoning packet
- 93% lean ground turkey, 1 pound
- A bag of mini sweet bell peppers

What You Do:

1. Start by halving the peppers and removing their seeds.
2. Set your oven to 350 degrees.
3. While the oven is heating up, brown the ground turkey.
4. Once the turkey is thoroughly cooked, drain off any fat that may have accumulated, and then sprinkle in the taco seasoning packet. Follow the directions on the packet for seasoning.
5. Place the halved bell peppers onto a baking sheet.
6. Ease the ground, seasoned turkey into the bell peppers.
7. Make sure you try to get an even amount of turkey into each bell pepper half.
8. Sprinkle the tops of each of the peppers with some cheese.

9. Place the baking tray in the oven and allow it to cook for five minutes.

10. Allow the peppers to cool slightly and then place over onto a serving plate.

11. Sprinkle them with cilantro and serve them with some salsa for dipping.

Calories: 210

Fat: 12.4 g

Protein: 17.9 g

Carb: 7 g

Roasted Corn Guacamole

Prep: 10 mins

Cook: 5 mins

Servings – 4-6

What You Need:

- Pepper,Salt
- Chili pepper, 1 tsp
- Garlic powder, 1 ½ tsp
- Chopped cilantro, ¼ cup
- Diced onion, ¼ cup
- Diced small tomato
- Lime juice, 2 tsp
- Large avocados, 2-3
- Cumin, 2 tsp, divided
- Butter, 1 tbs
- An ear of corn

What You Do:

1. Heat up a grill. Brush the corn with some butter and sprinkle it with a teaspoon of thecumin.

2. Lay the corn on the grill and cook it for five minutes. Make sure you turn it oftenduring the cooking process to make sure it browns evenly.

3. The corn should char slightly during the cooking process.

4. Take it off the grill, and with a sharp knife, slice off the

kernels. Set the kernels asideand discard the cob.

5. Pit the avocados and scoop out the meat of the avocados and place it in a bowl.

6. Mash up the avocados using a fork until they are creamy, but they still have a little bitof texture.

7. Mix in the garlic powder, chili powder, cilantro, and lime juice. Mix all of the ingredients together to make sure everything is evenly distributed.

8. Add in some pepper and salt to taste. Carefully stir in the corn, tomatoes, and onion.

9. Serve the guacamole immediately.

10. This is a great topper for any of the recipes in the beef and poultry sections of thisbook.

Calories: 189

Fat: 16.6 g

Protein: 2.7 g

Carb: 13.1 g

Bean and Spinach Burrito

Prep: 10 mins

Cook: 20 mins

Servings – 6

What You Need:

- Whole grain tortillas, 6
- Salt, to taste
- Fat-free Greek yogurt, 6 tbs
- Salsa, ½ cup
- Reduced-fat grated cheddar cheese, ½ cup
- Chopped romaine lettuce, ½ cup
- Cooked Mexican rice, 1 ½ cups
- Drained and rinsed black beans, 15 ounces
- Baby spinach, 6 cups

What You Do:

1. Set your oven to 300 degrees.

2. Stack all of the tortillas on top of each other and wrap them in a large piece ofaluminum foil.

3. Sit the stack of tortillas on a baking sheet and bake them for 15 minutes until heatedthrough.

4. Allow them to warm as you prepare the rest of the ingredients.

5. Add the spinach to the food processor and pulse it until they

are finely chopped. Ifyou don't have a food processor, you can also use a knife to slice up the leaves.

6. Place a large pan on medium heat and allow it to heat up.

7. Add in the spinach and black beans. Cook the mixture until the spinach has wilted. This should take around three minutes.

8. Evenly distribute this mixture between the six tortillas. Make sure that you leaveabout two inches on the end of the wrap to aid in folding it up.

9. Add about a quarter cup of the mixture to each tortilla and top with the lettuce, salsa,cheese, and the yogurt. Make sure you distribute the toppings evenly among them. Fold the tortilla over and under on the ends.

Calories: 371

Fat: 4.8 g

Protein: 14 g

Carb: 34 g

Stuffed Southwest Style Sweet Potatoes

Prep: 30 mins

Cook: 30 mins

Servings – 4

What You Need:

- Pepper
- Salt
- Chopped cilantro, 2 tbs
- Frozen corn kernels, ½ cup
- Ground cumin, 1 tsp
- Cooked black beans, ½ cup
- Chopped tomatoes with juices, 1 cup
- Chili powder, ½ tsp
- Diced red onion, 1 small
- Olive oil, 1 tsp
- Small sweet potatoes, 4
- Minced garlic, 1 clove

What You Do:

1. Set your oven to 400 degrees.
2. Sit the sweet potatoes on a cookie sheet and allow them to bake in your heated ovenfor 30 minutes.

3. Take the potatoes out of the oven and prick them a few times and then place themback in for another 30 minutes, or until they have become tender.

4. As the sweet potatoes are baking, place a pan on medium heat and allow it to heat up.

5. Add in the olive oil and the onions and allow them to cook for two minutes. Theonions should be soft, but they should not be translucent.

6. Add in the garlic and allow it to cook for 30 seconds or until you can start to smell thegarlic.

7. Mix in the salt, chili powder, and cumin. Mix everything together until well combined. Mix in the cilantro and season the mixture with a bit more pepper and salt.

8. Taste and adjust the flavorings as you need.

9. To serve the potatoes:

10. Take the sweet potatoes out of the oven and slice them down the middle.

11. Fluff the meat inside of the potato up a little and season it with a bit of salt.

12. Divide the filling you just made between the different potatoes.

13. Enjoy.

Calories: 224

Fat: 1.9 g

Protein: 8.4 g

Carb: 45.1 g

Vegetable Chili

Prep: 5 mins

Cook: 8 hrs

Servings – 12

What You Need:

- Cilantro, ½ cup
- Corn kernels, 1 cup
- Vegetable broth, 2 ½ cups
- Tomato paste, 6 ounces
- Diced green chilis, 4 ounces
- Cumin, 1 tsp
- Drained black beans, 2 cans
- Diced tomatoes, 2, 15-ounce cans
- Salt, 1 tsp
- Pepper, ½ tsp
- Diced sweet potato
- Diced celery, 1 cup
- Diced sweet onion, 1 cup
- Chili powder, 3 tbs
- Sliced carrots, 2 cups
- Dark red kidney beans, 1 can

What You Do:

1. Place all of the chili ingredients, except for the cilantro, into a slow cooker.

2. Stir everything together and place the lid on the cooker and then set it to cook for sixto eight hours on low.

3. Once it has finished cooking, sprinkle in the cilantro. You can also top the chili withsome diced avocado, sour cream, and shredded cheese.

Calories: 215

Fat: 1.5 g

Protein: 11 g

Carb: 45.2 g

Corn and Black Bean Salad

Prep: 30 mins

Cook: 0 mins

Servings – 6

What You Need:

- Pepper, ¼ tsp Olive oil, 2 tbs
- Dash of salt
- Brown sugar or honey, 1 tsp
- Minced garlic, 1 tsp
- Balsamic vinegar, ¼ cup
- Minced red onion, 2 tbs
- Chopped parsley, ¼ cup
- Drained and rinsed black beans, 2, 16-ounce cans
- Whole kernel corn, 1 cup

What You Do:

1. Place the parsley, red onion, black beans, and corn in a large bowl and mix everythingtogether.

2. Whisk the pepper, salt, honey, garlic, lemon juice, olive oil, and balsamic vinegartogether. Make sure that all of the seasonings are mixed together well.

3. Pour the dressing you just made over the corn and bean mixture.

4. Toss everything together and allow the vegetables to marinate for at least 30 minutesbefore you serve them.

5. This will allow all of the flavors to mix together, and the flavor will be a lot moreintense.

6. Enjoy

Calories: 155

Fat: 5.3 g

Protein: 3.4 g

Carb: 14.6 g

Spicy Peanut Vegetarian Chili

Prep: 10 mins

Cook: 40 mins

Servings – 10-12

What You Need:

- Vegetable broth, 2 cups
- Tomato sauce, 15 ounces
- Diced tomato, 28 ounces
- Powdered peanuts, ⅔ cup
- Rinsed and drained white beans, 16 ounces
- Rinsed and drained, black beans, 16 ounces
- Dried oregano, ¼ tsp
- Chipotle chili pepper, 1 tsp (optional)
- Chili powder, 2 tbs
- Minced garlic, 2 cloves
- Chopped onion, 1 cup
- Peanut oil, 1 tbs

What You Do:

1. In a Dutch oven, pour the oil in and let it heat up over medium-high heat.

2. Place in the onion and garlic and sauté them together for three to four minutes. Theonions should become tender, but make sure that you don't let your garlic burn.

3. Mix in the salt, oregano, pepper, and chili powder. Allow this mixture to sauté for another two minutes, or until it becomes fragrant.

4. Mix in the broth, tomato sauce, tomatoes, powdered peanuts, corn, and cleaned beans.

5. Stir everything together and let it all come to a boil.

6. Lower the heat down to a simmer and allow the mixture to cook for 30 minutes.

7. If you want, this can also be fixed in a slow cooker.

8. Add everything to the slow cooker and mix everything together.

9. Cover the slow cooker and set it to high for two to three hours.Calories: 96

Fat: 3.2 g

Protein: 6.8 g

Carb: 12.6 g

Black Bean, Rice, and Zucchini Skillet

Prep: 10 mins

Cook: 15 mins

Servings – 4

What You Need:

- Monterey Jack and Cheddar cheese blend, shredded, ½ cup
- Uncooked instant white rice, 1 cup
- Dried oregano, ¼ tsp
- Water, ¾ cup
- Undrained fire roasted diced tomatoes with garlic, 14.5 ounces
- Rinsed and drained black beans, 15 ounces
- Diced green bell pepper, ½ cup
- Chopped onion, ½ cup
- Small sliced zucchini
- Canola oil, 1 tbs

What You Do:

1. Start out by heating the oil in a large pan over medium heat.
2. Once it is well heated, add in the bell pepper, zucchini, and onion. Allow the veggiesto cook for five minutes, or until softened.
3. Make sure that you stir them occasionally.

4. Add in the oregano, water, undrained tomatoes, and beans.

5. Bring the heat up a bit and allow it to come to a boil.

6. Mix in the rice, stirring well to distribute all of the flavors.

7. Place the lid on the pan and then set it off the heat.

8. Allow the mixture to sit for seven minutes, or until the rice has absorbed all of thewater.

9. Sprinkle everything with cheese and enjoy.

Calories: 220

Fat: 8.4 g

Protein: 7.8 g

Carb: 28.7 g

Conclusion

As we draw to the close of 'Nourishing Recipes: A Gastric Sleeve Cookbook for Healthful Living,' we hope that you have found inspiration and guidance within its pages. Remember that your journey to healthful living doesn't stop here – it's a continual process of exploration and learning, full of rich tastes and discoveries.

This cookbook was created with the understanding that life after gastric sleeve surgery requires adaptability and patience, but that doesn't mean it has to be devoid of culinary pleasure. Whether you're in the early stages of your post-surgery diet or have fully transitioned to solid foods, the recipes in this book are designed to be a part of your long-term eating plan, contributing to a balanced and sustainable lifestyle.

Thank you for allowing us to accompany you on this journey. Remember, every meal is a step towards better health and wellbeing. Embrace the process, savor each bite, and always, happy cooking!

www.ingramcontent.com/pod-product-compliance
Lightning Source LLC
LaVergne TN
LVHW020813200726
843506LV00009B/1017